Lid Surgery—Current Concepts

Lid Surgery–
Current Concepts

Sidney A. Fox
M.S. (Ophth.) M.D., F.A.C.S.

Quondam Clinical Professor of Ophthalmology,
New York University School of Medicine;
Visiting Ophthalmologist, Bellevue Hospital;
Consultant Ophthalmologist, Bronx V.A. Hospital,
Goldwater Memorial Hospital,
Hospital for Joint Diseases and Medical Center
and St. Vincent's Hospital.

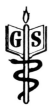

Grune & Stratton
New York and London

Library of Congress Cataloging in Publication Data

Fox, Sidney Albert, 1898–
  Lid surgery—current concepts.

  Includes bibliographies.
  1. Eyelids—Surgery. 2. Surgery, Plastic.
I. Title. [DNLM: 1. Eyelids—Surgery. 2. Surgery,
Plastic. WW 168 F794L 1972]
RE87.F58   617.7′71   72–4704
ISBN 0–8089–0774–3

Grune & Stratton, Inc.
111 Fifth Avenue
New York, New York 10003

Library of Congress Catalog Card Number 72-4704
International Standard Book Number 0-8089-0774-3
Printed in the United States of America

To My Patients

–To Whom Else?

Preface

*I speak truth, not so much as I would, but as much
as I dare, and I dare a little more as I grow older.*
—Montaigne

This is my eighth published volume and it comes closest—within the limitations of the above quotation—to being the book I have always wanted to write but which I have as yet not written.

I have tried to make it readable as well as informative. Ponderous and somnifacient writing is not necessarily profound, and simplicity often outdoes elegance in scientific accuracy. Hence I felt that the text would profit from an occasional lighter touch and a leavening historical tidbit. Some serious minded reviewers—those who actually read the text—may scoff at or be offended by an occasional light-minded phrase or quip, but I hope this will not be unwelcome to readers who expect the usual heavy tedium from a surgical textbook.

Max Planck once said that scientific progress is not made by rational, unemotional testing of theories but by having young men with better ideas replace old men who die off. Styles, ideas, and even basic philosophies are changing in this day of quarks, quesars, and tachyons. But, whatever the mechanism of change, one must maintain a sense of proportion among these multifarious innovations. New technics are not necessarily better technics and involved surgery is not always the most effective surgery despite recent embellishments and modifications. As much as possible I like to stick to fundamentals. It is easy to complicate a subject with theoretic considerations which are only peripherally germane to a basic theme.

Nor are current concepts necessarily new concepts. In fact, it is remarkable that so much basic ophthalmic plastic surgery has retained its validity and has remained unchanged. This is evidenced by the frequency with which "new" technics are found to have identical counterparts in the old literature—a coincidence that is sometimes truly wondrous. Thus procedures which were popular 100 and more years ago and later abandoned for good reason are rediscovered, brushed off, polished up, rechristened with new eponyms, and eased back into the literature.

This book contains the procedures I now prefer for most of the usual conditions requiring ophthalmic plastic surgery. It includes most of the worthwhile new surgical procedures of the past several years which have become current, important modifications of some older technics, and some of the fundamental operations which have withstood the test of time intact. Although it covers most of the important subjects of ophthalmic plastic surgery, it includes only one or two technics which I have found most useful for each condition. Hence although probably sufficiently inclusive to stand on its own, this book does not offer the multiple choices included in my preceding textbook. Its primary purpose therefore is to serve as a bridge between the fourth edition of *Ophthalmic Plastic Surgery* and, let us hope, a sometime future fifth edition.

The work of others has been attributed in all cases to the proper progenitors. Procedures which have been modified are so labeled; some are my own. A number of technics seem to be in the common domain of ophthalmic plastic surgery. In other words, their origins are shrouded in an obscurity which I have been unable to penetrate after reasonable search. Since my interest in historical origins is fairly well known, I should appreciate hearing of it if such information is available to anyone.

In a more or less serious vein, Ambrose Bierce once dedicated a book in quite in another context to those "enlightened souls who prefer dry wines to sweet, sense to sentiment, wit to humor and clean English to slang." I have neither Bierce's wit nor his wisdom, nor can I equal his felicity in the use of English. But I hope that those who prefer dry wines to sweet will understand and approve what I have tried to do here.

I am fortunate in having been able to retain my team of collaborators: Mrs. Helen Holoviak, critic and amanuensis; Mr. Lou Barlow, artist; and Mr. Walter S. Lentschner, photographer. It is not too much to say that they not only have eased my labors but have made this work possible.

Sidney A. Fox

Contents

CHAPTER 1

Basic Technics

The most important surgical characteristic of the human eyelid is its ability to withstand and survive almost any kind of traumatic insult short of complete destruction and still retain function and, very often, acceptable cosmetic appearance. This is due to several inherent factors peculiar to the lid:

1. Its superabundant vascular supply. We rarely have to worry where the blood supply is coming from. In fact, bleeding is often an embarrassment of riches.

2. Nerve supply—sensory and motor—is not a problem in lid repair and rarely necessitates pause for thought.

3. We like, when possible, to incise the lids horizontally, parallel with the course of the orbicularis fibers and the normal lid furrows, as this gives the best and most rapid healing and least visible scarring. But this is not always possible and the lids can withstand vertical, horizontal, and slanted incisions without any trouble and with good rapid healing.

4. The lids, both upper and lower, can stand a large percentage of tissue loss, especially skin—anywhere from 25 to 40 per cent, increasing with age—and still retain normal function and appearance.

5. This permits easy borrowing of portions of lid and the transfer of grafts from one lid to another—a tremendous advantage, since match of color and texture is perfect.

All these factors lend aid and comfort to our lid surgery and give us our ability to work our will with eyelids in many ways. For there are many technics for repairing lids, and in trained hands most work well. Few of these technics sprang full grown from the head of one genius. Most are the result of slow, sometimes painstaking, development in which numerous individuals had a hand.

SUTURES

It is difficult to think of surgery without sutures today. Yet it is only about 100 years since Lister showed that sutures could be sterilized and used without infecting the wound. Before this, most wounds were left to heal by "first intention" or granulation. Improvement in suture materials and needles followed rapidly and many excellent varieties are available. The sutures described below are those I have found most useful and have continued to use over the years.

Skin Wound Closure

LID SKIN SUTURES

The skin of the lid is so thin that interrupted sutures of 6-0 silk are usually adequate for adults. In infants and children, in whom postoperative suture removal is difficult, sometimes requiring anesthesia, 5-0 or 6-0 plain catgut will give a satisfactory closure.

EXTRAPALPEBRAL SUTURES

Beyond the lid and in a scarred lid, where the tissues are thicker, I prefer 5-0 silk and 4-0 catgut, respectively. In suturing the brow, where the skin is heavy indeed, I prefer 4-0 silk.

Sutures put in under some tension, even when wound edges have been mobilized maximally, should not be removed until healing is ensured. If suture removal is too early the scar may tend to widen and even become pigmented occasionally. This gives a cosmetically unacceptable scar which may require further surgery. Hence it is better to leave in sutures a day or two longer and incur the danger of suture marks which, in my experience, almost always absorb.

CHOICE OF SUTURE TECHNIC

When the lips of a wound fall together easily and without tension, a running suture, either cuticular (Fig. 1) or subcuticular (Fig. 2), gives a nice cosmetic and functional closure. These sutures may be locked at both ends to prevent loosening. If the wound gapes, a single interrupted or a continuous lock suture (Fig. 3), with the loops placed sufficiently close together to give complete closure, will work better.

Mattress sutures, both horizontal (Fig. 4) and vertical (Fig. 5) are indicated for relatively thicker tissues which close with some difficulty. They should take a deeper bite in the tissues and may be used in conjunction with interrupted shallower sutures. The continuous mattress suture (Fig. 6) is less useful here except that it avoids individual knotting and hence leaves fewer marks.

Deep mattress sutures should come out early, in 2 or 3 days. I do not hesitate to leave superficial skin sutures in 5 or even 6 days, as long as they are not under tension. Over many years I have found this quite satisfactory and have had little trouble from suture marks. It is far better to leave sutures in a day or two longer than to have wound lips spread and heal with a wide scar because sutures have been removed too early.

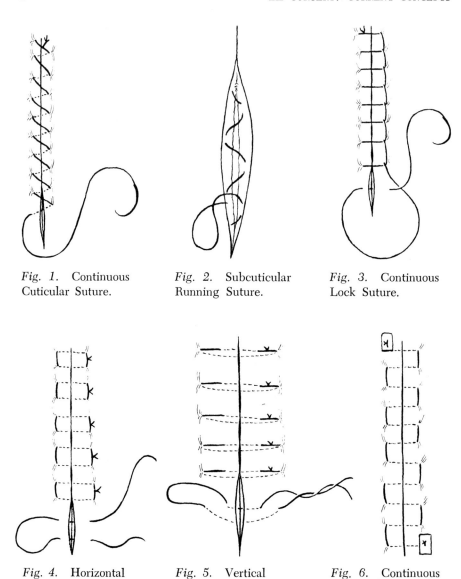

Fig. 1. Continuous Cuticular Suture.

Fig. 2. Subcuticular Running Suture.

Fig. 3. Continuous Lock Suture.

Fig. 4. Horizontal Mattress Suture.

Fig. 5. Vertical Mattress Suture.

Fig. 6. Continuous Mattress Suture.

Temporary Lid Closure

Suturing the upper and lower lids together is an important fundamental ophthalmic technic which needs no elaboration here. It splints the lids and reduces their movement to a minimum, thus aiding the healing process after lid repairs, reconstructions, skin grafting, and similar procedures. It provides an anatomic patch in cases of serious corneal pathology and is valuable in protecting the globe after orbital surgery and whenever prolonged pressure must be applied.

Under optimal conditions intermarginal sutures may be kept in from 10 to 20 days before reaction or infection sets in. However, they sometimes loosen or pull out before their function is fully accomplished. This may occur in lids whose vitality has been lowered by severe trauma or repeated surgical procedures. It may happen in lids narrowed congenitally or by loss of tissue due to trauma, or in severe exophthalmos with strong lid retraction. In all cases where the tendency to lid separation is so great that it jeopardizes the integrity of the intermarginal suture with or without tarsorrhaphy, I have found the following two technics rewarding in providing a lid union least likely to tear loose.

ORIGINAL FROST INTERMARGINAL SUTURE

The Frost suture as used today is considerably different from the one Frost originally described. In his technic the double-armed suture (Fig. 7) was passed through a peg and then through the skin below the ciliary margin to emerge through the gray line of the lower lid. The needles then pierced the opposing gray line of the upper lid as is done today. But Frost then continued his needles subcutaneously until they emerged above the brow where they were tied over a peg. This makes for a considerably firmer suture than the modified form now generally in use. Additionally, a horizontal spindle of skin was resected in the upper lid to prevent too much lid fold.

TARSAL BITE INTERMARGINAL SUTURE

The needles of a double-armed 4-0 silk suture are passed through a rubber peg. They are then entered into the skin of the lower lid about

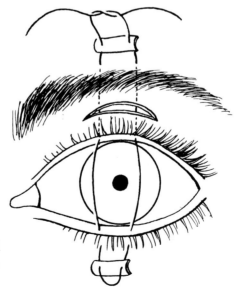

Fig. 7. Original Frost Intermarginal Suture. (From Frost, A. S. *Am. J. Ophthalmol.* 17:1633, 1934.)

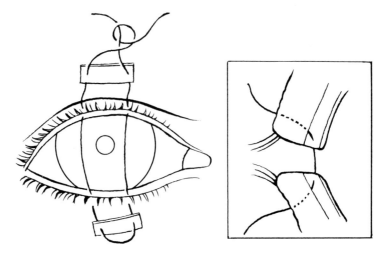

Fig. 8. Tarsal Bite Intermarginal Suture. Needles engage anterior surface of both tarsi (*inset*).

2 mm below the ciliary margin (Fig. 8). As the needles pass upward they engage the anterior surface of the tarsus before coming out on the lid border. As they enter the opposing upper lid they pass *behind* the gray line into the substance of the tarsus to emerge above the cilia of the upper lid (Fig. 8, *inset*), where they are tied over a peg.

Passing the sutures into the tarsal substance gives firmer anchorage to the intermarginal suture and a longer life span if it is needed.

Relaxation Sutures

Relaxation sutures are extremely helpful when tissue edges which must be brought together are under some tension. Their purpose is to reduce the surface skin tension by transferring some or all of it to the subcutaneous tissues, thus allowing relaxation of the skin. Such sutures are of special importance in advancing a pedicle flap forward into a desired position as seen in Figure 9. Of course, the pedicle must be completely undermined and well mobilized so that it is both free and under no tension. In lid repair there are at least two ways of using sutures to relax an advancement pedicle and ease it into required positions:

1. The subcutaneous suture of 4-0 or 5-0 catgut is inserted in the bed of the wound, then further back in the raw undersurface of the pedicle, so that when the suture is tied the pedicle is pulled forward in the direction of its desired position (Fig. 9A).

2. Lateral sutures are inserted first in the fixed tissues adjacent to the pedicle, then in the pedicle—again further back—so they are further forward in the fixed tissue than in the pedicle. When tied they pull the pedicle forward and advance its position (Fig. 9B).

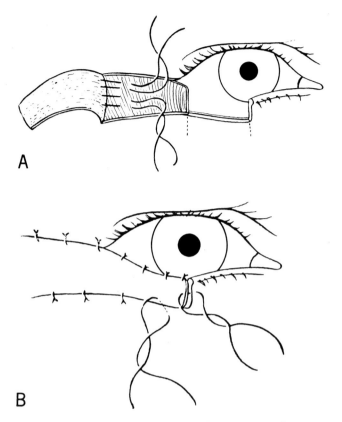

A

B

Fig. 9. Relaxation Sutures. *A.* Subcutaneous relaxation suture. *B.* Lateral relaxation skin suture. See text.

SURGICAL TARSORRHAPHIES

When prolonged closure of the lids is desired, surgical fusion (tarsorrhaphy) is needed. To counteract the tendency to stretch and narrow after a while, the through-and-through tarsorrhaphy has stood me well.

Through-and-Through Tarsorrhaphy—Author's Method

Surgical Technic (Fig. 10): The opposing lid margins are denuded of epithelium and split in the gray line shallowly in order to spread the margin and give more healing surface. Both needles of a double-armed 4-0 silk suture are passed through a rubber peg and then just below the ciliary margin, 4 mm apart, through the *full-thickness* of the lower lid

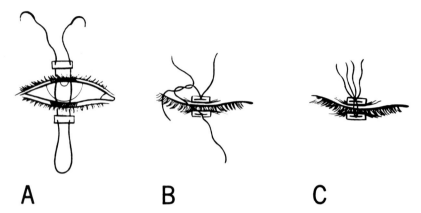

Fig. 10. Through-and-Through Tarsorrhaphy—Author's Technic. A. The opposing lid margins are denuded of epithelium for the desired length and split in the gray line shallowly to give more healing surface. A double-armed 4-0 silk suture is passed through a peg and then through the *full-thickness* lower lid just below the ciliary margin from skin to conjunctiva. It is similarly passed through the upper lid from within outward to emerge on the skin surface above the ciliary border and then through a peg. The needles are 4 mm apart. B. The lower loop is cut and the sutures tied. The needles are cut off and the upper sutures are tied so that the freshened areas of the lid margins come together. One of the upper sutures is being tied to one of the lower. C. Final appearance. (From Fox, S. A. *Arch. Ophthal.* 66:833, 1961.)

from skin to conjunctiva. They are then passed through the *full-thickness* of the opposing upper lid from conjunctiva to skin surface to emerge above the ciliary margin where they are passed through a peg again (Fig. 10A).

The lower suture loop is cut and the two ends are knotted over the lower peg and left long. The needles are cut off and the upper sutures tied so that the freshened opposing lid margins come together snugly (Fig. 10B). Each of the upper sutures is now firmly tied to one of the lower sutures (Fig. 10C) in order to equalize the anterior and posterior tension of the sutures on the lid margins and prevent buckling of the lid edges.

Comment: Since most surgical tarsorrhaphy sutures are passed through the gray line, piercing only the skin-muscle lamina of the lid, it is not surprising that they pull through when tissue vitality is low or when the tendency to lid separation is great. Pegs help but are no panacea because sutures can pull through, pegs and all. The above technic uses the full lid thickness, which includes the tough tarsal plates, and thus withstands tension pull much better. I have found this procedure especially useful in lids which have been operated on several times and as an accessory in advanced exophthalmos with lid retraction requiring lateral canthoplasty. In exophthalmos the wound edges of the lateral canthoplasty are in constant danger of pulling apart, and a reinforcing accessory intermarginal suture, placed medial to the canthoplasty, may mean the difference between surgical success and failure.

Tarsal Sliding Flap Tarsorrhaphy

An even firmer fusion which will last almost indefinitely is the tarsal sliding flap tarsorrhaphy. Here a little sliding graft of tarsoconjunctiva is used in a tongue-and-groove manner.

Surgical Technic (Fig. 11): The lids are pinched together and the margins are marked off. Both lids are then split within the marked-off limits, and vertical tarsoconjunctival incisions are made to create tongues of tarsoconjunctiva opposite each other in both lids. The tongue is resected from one lid to create a groove. The opposite slip of tarsoconjunctiva is dissected up and mobilized by further conjunctival incision and dissection so that there is no pull on the lid (Fig. 11). A double-armed 4-0 silk suture is passed through the edge of the tarsal slip from without inward. The needles are then passed through the upper edge of the opposing lid groove from within outward to emerge on the skin surface. The tarsal slip from the lower lid is thus pulled into the upper lid groove as the suture is tied over a peg. A firm dressing is applied to hold the tarsal tongue in position during healing.

Comment: This technic works equally well when the tongue and groove are transposed, i.e., when the tongue is fashioned in the upper lid and pulled into a lower lid groove. Like the through-and-through procedure, it is especially useful where the simpler tarsorrhaphies have failed. After

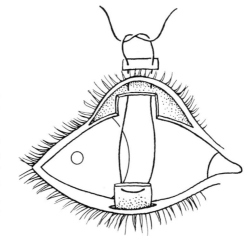

Fig. 11. Tarsal Sliding Flap Tarsorrhaphy. The upper and lower lids are split opposite each other. A tarsoconjunctival groove is fashioned in the upper lid and a tongue of tarsoconjunctiva in the lower lid. The tongue is drawn up into the groove with a double-armed suture, which is tied over a peg above the ciliary margin.

release it heals just as well as the simpler tarsorrhaphies. It is also more permanent and may be left in place much longer than the through-and-through tarsorrhaphy. However, since it requires somewhat more surgery and also tissue from an opposing lid, indications for the sliding flap procedure will probably not be as common as for the through-and-through tarsorrhaphy.

PLASTIES

Modification of Vertical Closure—Author's Method

Vertical scars in the lower lid are anathemas because of their tendency to pull the lower lid down and away from the globe, predisposing to ectropion. Hence any technic which modifies vertical closure of a

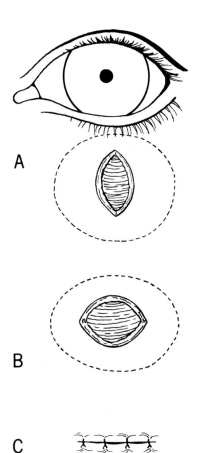

Fig. 12. Vertical Closure Modification —Author's Technic. A. Resection leaves a vertical spindle-shaped wound. This is completely undermined. B. The incision becomes rounded, and on further undermining the wound is pulled into a horizontal shape. C. Horizontal closure.

wound and swings it nearer to the horizontal is a welcome addition to the ophthalmic surgical armamentarium.

SIMPLE UNDERMINING

In small lesions of relaxed lower lids, usually in the elderly, it is sometimes possible to undermine the lips of the wound so completely that a vertical wound can be converted into a horizontal closure. It must be emphasized, however, that the wound must be small and the skin sufficiently atonic to permit this maneuver.

Surgical Technic (Fig. 12): When excision of a lesion leaves a vertical wound (Fig. 12A), the whole area is undermined completely, first into a round shape. Then, if the skin is sufficiently lax, the wound is pulled into a horizontal spindle shape (Fig. 12B) and closed horizontally (Fig. 12C).

VARIABLE WOUND LIP UNDERMINING

In larger lesions it is possible to swing a slanted line of closure into a more horizontal position by careful and variable undermining of the wound lips, modifying downward pull of the lid and avoiding ectropion. Again this requires a rather lax atonic skin such as is found in an older individual. Also the lesion resected must be not too large and not too vertical.

Surgical Technic (Fig. 13): When excision of a lesion (Fig. 13A) leaves a more vertical than horizontal wound, the medial half of the upper wound lip and the lateral half of the lower wound lip are undermined (Fig. 13B). On closure, the medial half of the upper wound lip is pulled down and the lateral half of the lower wound lip pulled up (Fig. 13C). The closed wound thus assumes a much more horizontal position (Fig. 13D) and exerts relatively little downward pull on the lower lid. Figure 13E shows the final result.

Flat-X Plasty—Author's Method

A large extramarginal lid wound created by resection of a round, rectangular, or irregular lesion would require the sacrifice of tissue for conversion into a horizontal spindle for easier closure. This would be especially undesirable in the case of obviously benign lesions. Is such cases the following simple plasty has been found useful.

Surgical Technic (Fig. 14): After resection of the lesion an incision is made continuing the lower lip of the wound in an upward curve to form flap A. Flap B is similarly formed by continuing the upper lip of the wound downward on the other side. The pointed tips of the flaps are

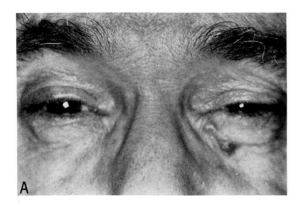

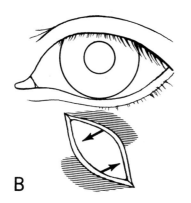

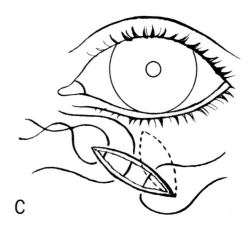

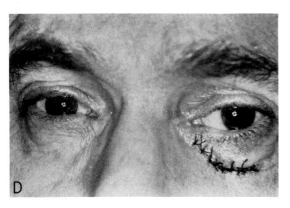

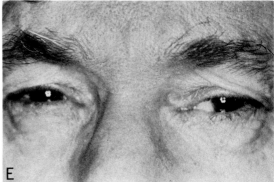

Fig. 13. Change of Wound Closure Direction—Author's Technic. *A.* Neoplasm below left lower lid. *B.* After lesion is resected, the medial half of the upper wound lip and the lateral half of the lower wound lip are undermined. *C.* and *D.* On closure the upper lip is pulled down and the lower lip up. The wound is now in a more horizontal position. *E.* Final result.

Fig. 14. Flat-X Plasty—Author's Technic. *A.* After resection of the lesion, the upper and lower wound lips are extended downward and upward, respectively, on opposite sides. *B.* The resultant flaps are mobilized, the tips are resected, and the ends sutured together. *C.* The wound lips are undermined and closure made with interrupted sutures. (From Fox, S. A. *Arch. Ophthalmol.* 72:204, 1965.)

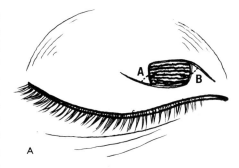

A

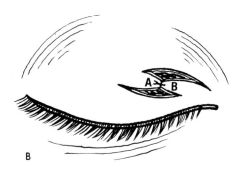

B

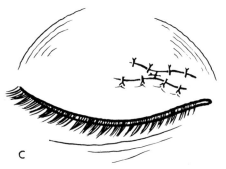

C

resected for easier suturing (Fig. 14A). The flaps A and B are undermined and mobilized so they can be advanced centrally and the tips sutured. This converts the original wide wound into two narrow horizontal wounds (Fig. 14B). The edges are undermined sufficiently to permit suturing (Fig. 14C).

Z Plasty

The Z plasty is an old and simple technic used to reduce skin pull in one direction at the expense of another, usually perpendicular to it, or nearly so. It is especially valuable in tissue areas that are sufficiently elastic to permit stretching and transposition of pedicles, which are not necessarily of identical size, by supplying tissue from one area to another. Thus by allowing transfer of tissue from one area to another the Z plasty may be used to (1) relieve tension and (2) supply tissue.

Surgical Technic (Fig. 15): If there is tension due to tissue contraction along the vertical line *bc* and it is desired to reduce this tension, the Z figure is incised as shown in Figure 15A. There are now two triangular flaps, *abc* and *bcd*, based on line *bc*. It will be noted that the distance *ad* is longer than *bc*. After the flaps *abc* and *bcd* have been dissected up and transposed (Fig. 15B), the figure assumes the form seen in Figure 15C. Triangle *abc* becomes *adc* and *bcd* becomes *bad*.

Thus *bc* is now longer than *ad*, and the amount of relaxation along line *bc* is the difference in length between *bc* and *ad* in the original figure. The angles *abc* and *bcd* should be less than 50° or it will be difficult to transpose the flaps unless the skin is unusually thin and extensible. The angles need not be equal to each other; some situations require one angle smaller than the other. The disparity in size may be as much as 20° but not more.

Modified Z Plasty

In a useful modification of the Z plasty the wound of excision forms the upper or lower horizontal arm of the Z.

Surgical Technic (Fig. 16): After excision of the neoplasm two pedicle flaps are formed by making incisions *cd* and *ef* (Fig. 16A). The flap *bcd* is undermined and pulled over so that *c* lies at *a*. The wound is

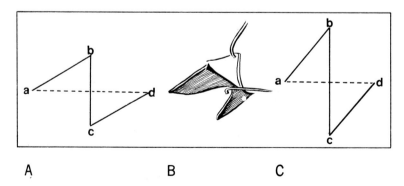

A   B   C

Fig. 15. Z Plasty. *A.* The Z incision *abcd*. *B.* Flaps are raised and mobilized. *C.* Result of transposition. Note that *bc* is now longer than *ad*.

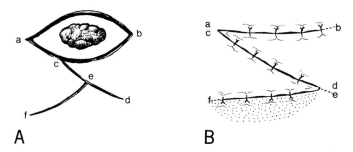

Fig. 16. Modified Z Plasty. *A.* The lesion is resected, and incisions *cd* and *ef* are made. *B.* The wound *ab* is closed, and flaps *bcd* and *cef* are undermined, mobilized, and sutured at *a* and *d*, respectively.

closed horizontally along the line *ab*. The pedicle *def* is then undermined similarly and pulled over so that *e* rests at *d*, completing the Z figure (Fig. 16*B*).

Comment: It will be noted that the flaps are not transposed. This procedure suffices for the average case. Sometimes when the area to be closed is large, the incisions have to be extended somewhat (dotted lines). Also the tissue below *ef* may have to be undermined to permit easy closure.

BASIC AUXILIARY TECHNICS

There are a few minor but basic technics which have been in the ophthalmologist's surgical armamentarium for many years and which have stood him well. Among these are the twins, canthotomy and cantholysis, used for lid relaxation, and Burow's clever little triangle for flattening out skin wrinkles. Their routine—almost automatic—use belies their undoubted importance: Ophthalmic surgery would be poorer without them. They frequently make the difference between a smooth, simply obtained, good cosmetic and functional result and one which would have been more difficult to attain without them. Hence, old or new, they must be included in any discussion of basic technics.

Canthotomy and Cantholysis

Canthotomy needs no introduction to ophthalmologists. It is an old friend long used to diminish lid pressure on the globe, as in cataract, glaucoma, proptosis, etc.

Cantholysis is a less frequently used maneuver in which the upper or lower arm of the lateral canthal ligament is lysed after canthotomy. This gives an additional relaxation of 4 or 5 mm to the involved lid and facilitates the closing of a coloboma whose lips might otherwise be under tension.

Surgical Technic (Figs. 21B and 25B): A lateral canthotomy is made in the usual fashion. After cessation of hemorrhage the arms of the canthal ligament are put on stretch and separated. The conjunctival lip of the wound is grasped with forceps, and the white arm of the cut ligament identified. The scissors are inserted to straddle the ligament, which is then cut with one stroke. When this is done the lid is felt to "give" under the fingers. No sutures are necessary as healing is uncomplicated and uneventful.

Burow's Triangle

This triangle first saw the light of day in 1838. It is a most useful technic which has smoothed away many a skin wrinkle since. Its effective use is shown in Chapter 2, Figure 18.

REFERENCES

Fox, S. A. New tarsorrhaphy suture. *Arch. Ophthal.* 66:833, 1961.
Fox, S. A. The flat-X plasty. *Arch. Ophthal.* 72:204, 1965.
Frost, A. D. Supportive suture in ptosis operation. *Am. J. Ophthalmol.* 17:1633, 1934.

CHAPTER 2

Lid Repairs

Ophthalmic plastic surgery reached what appeared to be its full development when the late John Wheeler returned from abroad with the vast surgical experience he had gained in the First World War. He gave us lid halving and lid splitting and popularized the free skin graft which ophthalmologists had been slow in adopting. These technics dominated ocular adnexal surgery for almost three decades until the early 1950's when new procedures slowly began to replace them. These changes are still in progress. They are not as dramatic as heart surgery or as startling as organ transplants—but their effect is as certain. One has only to compare books published in the last few years with those of 15 and 20 years ago to note the innovations that have taken place. The general tendency has been to simplify.

The most important and fundamental change, perhaps, is the gradual abandonment of lid halving and splitting in lid repairs. Since these two technics usually complement each other, it is no surprise that they should fade out at the same time. There are several reasons for this. Lid halving is an extravagant technic calling for the unnecessary sacrifice of normal tissue; lid splitting jeopardizes cilia. But a more important reason is that a better technic has been found to replace both—the intermarginal or figure-8 suture. The figure-8 suture has undergone many modifications since first reported by Minsky, but essentially it consists of full-thickness wound closure and splinting one lid to the opposing lid to prevent movement and thus hasten the healing process. This has taken the place of the halving procedure to a large extent.

The gradual abandonment of lid halving has resulted in another interesting development—the use of the same repair technics for ciliary margin and full margin lesions. Obviously the resection of a full-thickness wedge by the figure-8 technic when only the ciliary margin is involved means the sacrifice of healthy tissue. But the justification for this is unanswerable: The procedure is easier to do and gives a better result.

Figure-8 Splinting Suture—Minsky's Method (Modified)

The Minsky suture is best used for lesions which are perpendicular to the lid margin or reasonably so. I have modified and simplified it from Minsky's original reported technic.

18

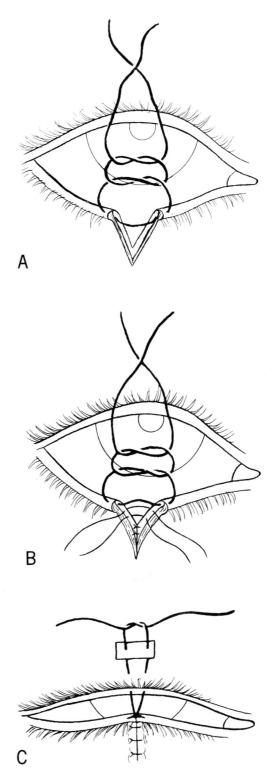

Fig. 17. Intermarginal (figure-8) Suture—Minsky's Procedure (Modified). A. The intermarginal suture is placed and double-knotted, but not tied. B. The tarsoconjunctiva is sutured from behind forward with suture knots on the anterior tarsus. C. The intermarginal suture is passed into the upper lid and tied, and the skin is sutured.

Surgical Technic (Fig. 17): After suitable infiltration anesthesia one needle of a double-armed 4-0 silk suture is entered in the gray line 3 mm from one side of the lid break to emerge in the wound about 4 mm below the lid margin. The needle is entered in the opposite lip of the wound, again 4 mm below the margin, to emerge in the gray line 3 mm from the edge of the laceration. The two arms of the suture are crossed to check on the alignment of the wound lips and make sure there is no vertical or horizontal displacement. The suture is double-knotted but not tied (Fig. 17A). The lid is pulled forward by means of this suture, and the tarsoconjunctiva is closed with 5-0 or 6-0 interrupted chromic catgut sutures as necessary. It will be noted that the tarsoconjunctiva is sutured in front so that the knots lie on the anterior tarsal surface and are later buried (Fig. 17B). This is the most important layer of sutures since the tarsus is the only firm, skeleton-like structure which gives the lid its shape, firmness, and rigidity. The marginal suture is tied and the needles passed through the gray line of the *opposing* lid to emerge in the skin above the ciliary margin, where they are tied over a peg. The skin wound in the lower lid is closed with 5-0 interrupted silk sutures (Fig. 17C). Healing is usually uneventful and the skin sutures are removed on the fifth or sixth day. The marginal suture in the tarsus is left in for 9 or 10 days unless it loosens earlier.

Comment: This suture works equally well for upper or lower lid lacerations. Placing the knots on the anterior surface of the tarsus avoids corneal abrasion if the lid break is near the cornea. Also if the lid is shortened and edematous, eversion to permit insertion of the conjunctival sutures may be difficult; placing them from in front in such cases is easier. After the tarsoconjunctiva is sutured, the intermarginal suture is completed and the skin sutures inserted.

The figure-8 suture has a double function: (1) to close the marginal wound and (2) to prevent notching. It is easy enough to suture a marginal wound as long as the lips can be brought together easily; the trick is to prevent notching. The figure-8 does this in two ways:

1. By creating a marginal pucker as the suture is tied. For this a stout 4-0 silk suture should be used and the *primary* loop should be in the lid margin. Two or three lighter weight sutures will not do, nor will a double-loop suture of which the first loop is buried in the depths of the wound. Such a loop anchors the figure-8 suture below the margin and does not permit the flexibility at the margin which causes the wound lips to pucker upward.

2. By using the opposing lid as a splint or anchor to exert vertical pull, thus counteracting lateral pull of the orbicularis. This splinting feature may not always be necessary, especially if tissue loss is small and the wound shallow. But in deep wounds notching is a constant possibility. So little time is needed to unite the two lids that the effort is well worthwhile in all cases to avoid notching in only a few.

The figure-8 is a versatile technic, useful in both small and large lid lesions. When employed in conjunction with canthotomy and cantholysis a sliding flap may even be added. The figure-8 method not only saves tissue but spares cilia, which are often lost during a halving procedure.

Temporal Advancement Flap with Burow's Triangle

The importance of the temporal advancement flap in modern lid surgery cannot be overestimated. It is described here not because it is unusual or new, but because it is a fundamental technic used either alone or in combination with other methods of lid repair and reconstruction, especially canthotomy and cantholysis. A glance at the procedures described in Chapter 3 makes this clear.

Obviously its main importance is in the handling of lesions involving the temporal half of the lid, for here advantage can be taken of the wide-open spaces of the temporal region to form an advancement pedicle to fill in a lid dehiscence due to trauma or tumor resection (Fig. 18A). Like the figure-8 suture, the advancement flap can be used for smaller lesions and in combination with other technics for larger repairs (Figs. 21, 22, 25, etc.).

Surgical Technic (Fig. 18): As the flap is advanced medially, the fixed tissue to each side and behind is frequently thrown in folds owing to the pull of the pedicle. These wrinkles and folds may smooth out spontaneously in time. However, it is better not to count on it. Burow showed how simple it is to smooth out the fixed tissues by resecting small triangles with the apex away from the pedicle.

The area of puckered skin (Fig. 18A) is included in a triangular incision with the apex pointing away from the line of repair (Fig. 18B).

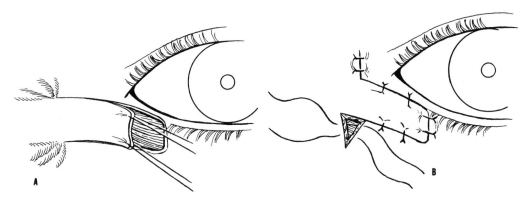

Fig. 18. Temporal Advancement Flap with Burow's Triangle. *A.* A temporal advancement flap is fashioned for repair of the lateral portion of the lid. *B.* Burow's triangle is resected on each side and closed.

The pucker is eliminated by a simple linear closure which is perpendicular to the major line of closure.

Modified (Indirect) Halving at Lower Punctum—Author's Method

It was stated above that the halving technic is on the way out. This is true. But the modified type of halving described here is one of the few technics that seems uniquely adapted to the unusual lesion that involves the area anterior to the lower punctum, but not the punctum itself (Fig. 19A). If such a lesion is not too large, this type of repair may save the lacrimal drainage apparatus where no other technic will.

Surgical Technic (Fig. 19): The lid in the region of the punctum is carefully split into its two laminae and the split is extended laterally for several millimeters (Fig. 19B). The lesion in front of the punctum is carefully dissected away in a triangular fashion. At the lateral end of the lid split a wedge of tarsoconjunctiva is resected (Fig. 19C).

The tarsoconjunctiva is closed with 5-0 chromic catgut sutures tied on the anterior tarsal surface. The skin-muscle wound is closed with 5-0 silk on the anterior surface and a couple of 6-0 sutures on the margin (Fig. 19D). Appearance of the repair before removal of sutures is seen in Figure 19E and the final result in Figure 19F.

Comment: Resection and suture of healthy tarsus helps shorten the lid and brings the edges of the skin-muscle wound closer together. This makes for easier closure and less lid splitting, thus avoiding more possible cilia loss.

Tumor Removal

The lid malignancies with which nature rewards the adult and the elderly continue to be the subject of interest in recent ophthalmic literature. The ratio of benign to malignant neoplasms varies as usual with each report, as does the frequency of recurrence after the use of the various modalities of tumor extirpation: surgery, x-ray, cryotherapy, and chemosurgery. Surgery does seem to have the edge in permanent cures as compared with irradiation. Cryotherapy and chemosurgery are new technics which have recently entered the lists of tumor therapy.

Whatever modality is used, knowledge that a neoplasm has been completely extirpated is of critical importance and can never be gauged by appearance alone. Two recent studies suggest that additional surgery should not be undertaken hastily if a tumor is reported incompletely excised because, according to these reports, only about one-third actually recur (Einaugler and Henkind). However, this is cold comfort when the one

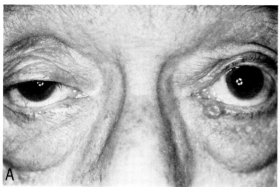

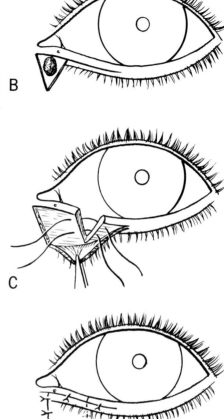

Fig. 19. Modified Halving at Lower Punctum—Author's Technic. *A.* Neoplasm anterior to left lower punctum. *B.* The lid behind the lesion is split and the split is carried laterally. The lesion is resected triangularly. *C.* The lid split is deepened and a wedge of tarsoconjunctiva, apex-down, is resected laterally. Conjunctival sutures are placed. *D* and *E.* The tarsoconjunctiva is closed on the anterior tarsal surface (dotted line) and the skin sutured. *F.* Final result. (From Fox, S. A. *Ophthalmic Plastic Surgery*, ed. 4. New York, Grune & Stratton, 1970.)

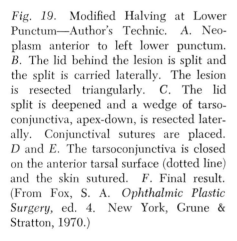

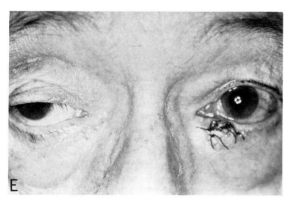

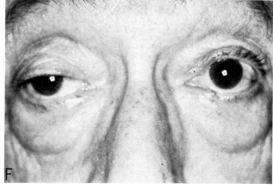

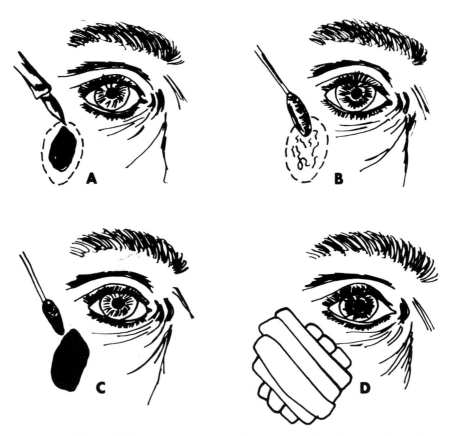

Fig. 20. Technic of Chemosurgery. *A.* The lesion is outlined. *B.* A keratolytic agent is applied to increase absorption. *C.* Zinc chloride paste is applied. *D.* The area is covered with an occlusive dressing. *E.* The fixed tissue is removed en bloc and mapped. *F.* The specimens are examined by frozen section. *G.* (*opposite page*) The fixative is reapplied to areas still showing cancer cells. (From Robins, P. In S. A. Fox (ed.). *Ophthalmic Plastic Surgery*, ed. 4. New York, Grune & Stratton, 1970.)

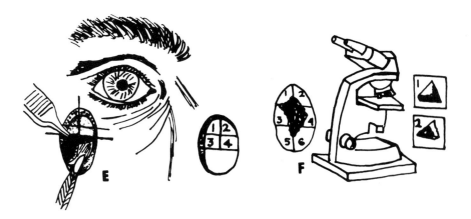

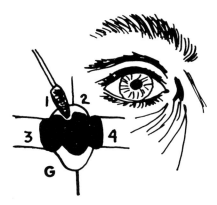

out of three does pop up. The decision to reoperate will also depend on the type of tumor, its malignancy, and its propensity to metastasize. Recent suggestions have included (1) geographic localization of the tumor edges and (2) separate resection of the wound edges after tumor excision in order to determine what edge needs further surgery if tumor tissue has not been removed completely. It is difficult to understand why the second step is necessary if the tumor edges have been properly identified initially.

Recently two new modalities—cryosurgery and chemosurgery—have been suggested for the cure of lid neoplasms. Cryotherapy uses liquid nitrogen and chemosurgery uses an escharotic paste. It has been shown that freezing a cell does not guarantee its destruction and that some survive. Hence chemosurgery seems to offer greater assurance of complete extirpation of a neoplasm.

CHEMOSURGERY

The advantage of chemosurgery is not the method itself, which is cumbersome, repetitive, and prolonged. Its advantage lies in the technic used to assure complete removal of the tumor. (I am not referring here to the type of facial chemosurgery done primarily with phenol mixtures for the eradication of skin wrinkles. This I leave to cosmetic surgeons.)

As with all destructive modalities, such as x-ray and cryotherapy, chemosurgery may be used interchangeably with surgery in small lesions with about equally good results. However, in large lesions which require repair afterward, surgery is by far the better method, as repair can usually be done at once without subjecting the patient to more than one trip to the operating room. The area of ophthalmic plastic surgery where chemosurgery is most useful is in the handling of large infiltrating lesions in the nasocanthal angle. These lesions penetrate deeply, sometimes to the lacrimal sac and periosteum. Usually it is almost impossible to remove them intact. Here then, if anywhere, diagnosis of complete extirpation is a critical necessity, and the method of examination described below becomes valuable.

Chemosurgery Technic (Fig. 20): After the lesion is outlined (Fig. 20A) a keratolytic agent such as dichloracetic acid is applied to the lesion to increase its percutaneous absorption. This coagulates the epidermal proteins and gives them a whitish color (Fig. 20B). Then a thin layer of 40 per cent zinc chloride paste in stilbinite is applied (Fig. 20C). This usually penetrates the tissues to a depth of 2 mm. The area is covered by an occlusive dressing to prevent the paste from liquefying and to assure complete penetration of the paste (Fig. 20D).

In 24 hours the fixed tissue is removed en bloc, marked with dye, and sectioned into 1-cm pieces according to a map which marks the origin and size of each piece (Fig. 20E). While the patient waits, all the cut specimens are examined by frozen section (Fig. 20F). If a specimen edge shows residual cancer cells, it is assumed that adjacent tissue also will, and the fixative is reapplied to the particular area or areas in which the tumor cells were found (Fig. 20G).

Thus only those areas which show incomplete removal of tumor cells are subjected to further treatment. The procedure is repeated until the whole area is cancer-free. Usually a layer of fixed tissue remains, which is sloughed, and the area is then allowed to granulate if it is small; if large, reparative surgery must be done. The 5-year cure rate of this modality is something over 90 per cent.

As stated above, for the ophthalmologist this chemosurgical technic would seem to be of most value for deep infiltrating lesions, especially in the nasocanthal angle where the medial canthal ligament and even the lacrimal sac may be involved. It is difficult to find a line of demarcation in this area, and the malignancy, not being compact, has to be removed piecemeal. The examination of serial frozen sections is of significant assistance in assuring complete tumor removal.

REFERENCES

Aurora, A. L., and Blodi, F. C. Reappraisal of basal cell carcinoma of the eyelids. *Am. J. Ophthalmol.* 70:329, 1970.

Burow, A. Zur Blepharoplastik. *Monatsschr. Med. Augenheilkd. Chir.* 1:57, 1838.

Cole, J. G. Controlled excision of eyelid tumors. *Am. J. Ophthalmol.* 70:240, 1970.

Einaugler, R. B., and Henkind, P. Basal cell epithelioma of the eyelid. *Am. J. Ophthalmol.* 67:413, 1969.

Gooding, C. A., White, G., and Yatsuhashi, M. Significance of marginal extension of basal cell carcinoma. *N. Engl. J. Med.* 273:923, 1965.

Lommatsch, P., Vollmer, R., and Lommatsch, K. The five-year cure rate of malignant lid tumors after radiation therapy. *Klin. Monatsbl. Augenheilkd.* 154:486, 1969.

Minsky, H. Surgical repair of recent lid lacerations: Intermarginal splinting suture. *Surg. Gynecol. Obstet.* 75:449, 1942.

Robins, P. Chemosurgery. In S. A. Fox, *Ophthalmic Plastic Surgery*, ed. 4, New York, Grune & Stratton, 1970, chap. 26.

Wilder, L. W., and Smith, B. Determination of the tumor margin in the excision of basal cell epitheliomas of the eyelids. *Ann. Ophthalmol.* 2:887, 1970.

Zacarian, S. A. The cryogenic approach to treatment of lid tumors. *Ann. Ophthalmol.* 2:706, 1970.

CHAPTER 3

Lid Reconstruction

The use of huge advancement and rotated pedicle flaps for lid reconstruction probably goes back to antiquity and certainly to the late Middle Ages. Until 100 years ago ophthalmic plastic surgery—indeed all plastic surgery—was based on the universally accepted dictum of Gasparo Tagliacozzi: "In order to live, a graft must have an attachment. It cannot be completely severed from the surrounding tissues. It must have a pedicle." Thus eye surgeons were limited to the huge advancement and rotated skin flaps described in early ophthalmology textbooks.

Then in 1870 the whole concept of skin grafting changed almost overnight. First Reverdin reported his epoch-making work on the transplantation of free pinch grafts. He was followed in short order by Lawson (1870), Le Fort (1872), Ollier (1872), Thiersch (1874), Sichel (1875), and Wolfe (1876), all of whom showed that free skin grafts—small and large, split-skin and full-thickness—could live and thrive in distant beds separated from their local blood supply.

Once there was no need for the giant rotated flaps with their mighty scars, ophthalmic plastic surgery gradually evolved new technics. This did not occur all at once—old habits do not fade easily in the medical world—but over the years ocular adnexal surgery slowly took on a character of its own. Attached grafts were not wholly abandoned. On the contrary, they were adapted, refined, and incorporated into procedures more suitable to the finer, less gross requirements of the lid surgery we know today. A few of these procedures are described below. Some have been known and used for years; others are so new that ophthalmic literature has not yet caught up with their importance or assessed their value.

Temporal Advancement Flap

PRIMARY INDICATION: *Loss of lateral half of upper or lower lid*

The oldest and probably simplest of reconstructive technics is the temporal advancement flap for lateral lesions of the upper or lower lid. It is of basic importance because it is used in combination with many of the other technics described below (e.g., Figs. 22, 23, 25, 29). The temporal region offers ample room and tissue for such a flap, which can be raised without injury to its surroundings. This is a much more convenient place for lid repair than the nasocanthal area, with its tear drainage channels and more constricted nasocanthal angle. Unfortunately, neoplasms occur more frequently medially than temporally.

Surgical Technic (Fig. 21): The flat, rodent tumor seen in the right lower lid (Fig. 21A) is resected including the lateral half of the lid. A canthotomy is performed, the lower arm of the ligament severed, and an advancement flap of skin is outlined laterally (Fig. 21B). The flap is raised and advanced medially by means of subcutaneous relaxation sutures (Fig. 21C). (See Chapter 1 for discussion of relaxation sutures.) The conjunctival edge of the wound is undermined, mobilized, drawn up, and sutured to the medial and lateral edges of the wound, thus completing repair of the lower fornix (Fig. 21C, *inset*). The advancement flap is sutured medially and below to the fixed medial portion of the lid and to the conjunctival margin (Fig. 21D). Figure 21E shows the lid before suture removal and Figure 21F shows the final result.

Comment: It is easier sometimes to suture the conjunctiva to the back of the skin flap before the flap is moved into position. Both the upper and lower lids are equally amenable to such repair, and half a lid can usually be reconstructed satisfactorily with the addition of canthotomy and cantholysis, as shown here.

Full-Thickness Lid Grafts

PRIMARY INDICATION: *Loss of half or more of upper or lower lid*

Lid reconstruction by means of full-thickness grafts from one lid to another, only recently experimental, has earned a permanent and useful place in opthalmic plastic surgery. I have done such grafting from one upper lid to another, from one lower lid to another, from an upper to a lower lid, and from a lower to an upper lid. All have done well and, indeed, seem to heal better and more rapidly than the plain free skin grafts. It was originally introduced by Callahan and more recently by Youens in 1967. The technic of full thickness grafting can be used for all lesions involving half or more of the upper or lower lid.

LOSS OF HALF A LID

The procedure described below illustrates transfer of a full-thickness graft from the left lower lid to the right lower lid. The patient had a neoplasm involving the whole punctal area of the right lower lid (Fig. 22A).

Surgical Technic (Fig. 22): After suitable anesthesia—I prefer local where possible—the lesion is resected in toto with a 4-mm margin of normal tissue all around. (The resected segment was 15 mm long and 8 mm wide.) A canthotomy of the right lateral canthus is made and the

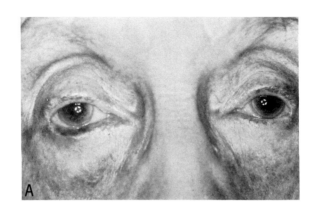

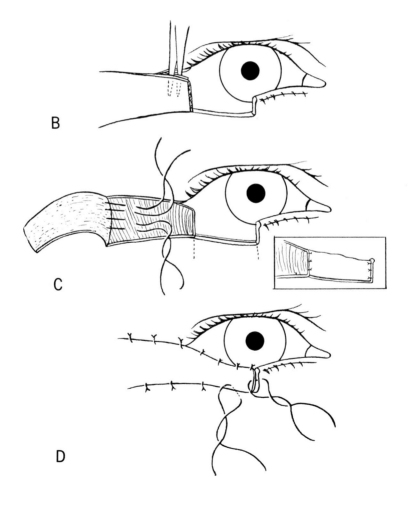

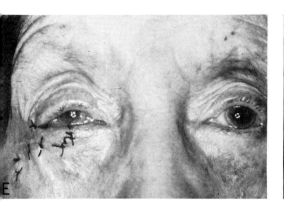 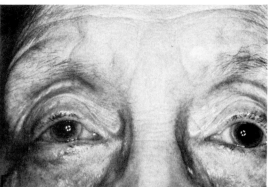

Fig. 21. Repair by Temporal Advancement Flap. *A. (opposite page)* Flat marginal tumor of the lateral right lower lid. *B. (opposite page)* The tumor is resected. Canthotomy and cantholysis are done and a temporal flap is outlined. *C. (opposite page)* A vertical conjunctival flap is mobilized (dotted lines), pulled up, and sutured *(inset)*. The skin flap is then advanced medially with the help of relaxation sutures. *D. (opposite page)* The skin flap is sutured into position and to the conjunctival flap at the margin. *E.* Appearance before suture removal. *F.* Final result.

lower arm of the canthal ligament cut. This allows mobilization of the lower lid and reduction of the dehiscence to 10 mm without the fashioning of an advancement flap (Fig. 22B). The conjunctiva, however, may have to be pulled up and readjusted laterally (Fig. 22C). By prolonging the canthotomy incision laterally through skin and orbicularis and undermining, additional mobility is obtained when necessary (Fig. 22B, dotted line).

A 12-mm full-thickness graft is taken at the lateral canthus of the left lower lid and sewed into the dehiscence in the right lower lid (Fig. 22D and F). The suturing is done with 6-0 chromic catgut on the conjunctival side and 5-0 silk sutures on the skin side. It is important to catch up *all* the layers of both graft and host in the sutures. This is especially true of the muscle layer from which the graft derives much of its blood supply.

Canthotomy and cantholysis of the lower arm of the ligament are done at the left lateral canthus and an advancement flap is fashioned. The cut end of the conjunctiva is undermined, pulled up, and sutured medially and laterally to the cut edges (Fig. 22E). The advancement flap is mobilized by undermining and drawn over to close the surgical coloboma in the left lower lid (Fig. 22F). The eyes are patched. No pressure dressing is necessary since there is no vascular bed. The graft gets its nourishment from the three cut edges only.

The sutures are removed from the left (donor) lid on the sixth day and the right (recipient) lid on the tenth day. The postoperative condition of the grafted lid 2 months later is shown in Figure 22G.

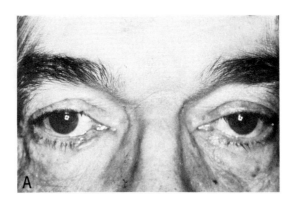

Fig. 22. Full-Thickness Graft Repair for Loss of Half a Lid—Youens' Method (Modified). *A.* Neoplasm of the medial half of the right lower lid. *B.* The tumor is resected. Right canthotomy and cantholysis of the lower arm of the canthal ligament are done. The skin incision may have to be prolonged laterally (dotted line) for increased lid mobility. *C.* The conjunctiva is pulled up, readjusted, and sutured at the margin (if necessary). *D.* A graft, taken from the left lower lid, is sewed into the right lower lid dehiscence. *E.* Canthotomy and cantholysis are performed, a temporal flap is made in the left lower lid, and the conjunctiva is pulled up. *F.* (*opposite page*) Appearance of both lids on completion of repair. *G.* (*opposite page*) Final result.

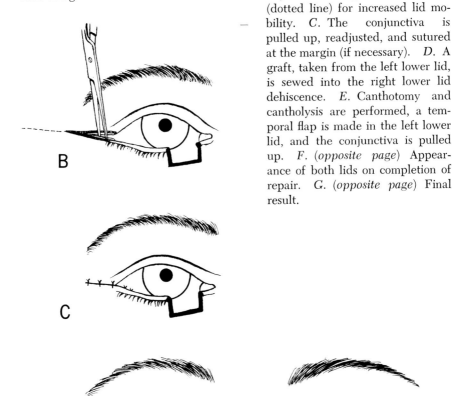

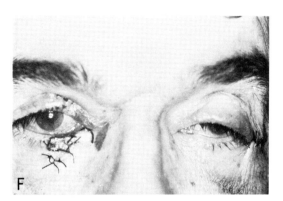
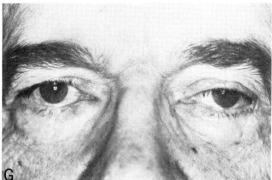

LOSS OF MORE THAN HALF A LID

When more than half a lid must be replaced, the procedure becomes a bit more complicated and requires not only a full-thickness graft from another lid but help from the all-purpose and always useful temporal advancement graft. The patient shown in figure 23A lost most of his left lower lid as a result of too enthusiastic an application of cautery for senile entropion. Repair was made by means of an advancement graft from the temporal region plus a full-thickness graft from the ipsilateral upper lid.

Surgical Technic (Fig. 23): A left lateral canthotomy is made and both arms of the canthal ligament are lysed. A lower lid pedicle flap is fashioned temporally (Fig. 23B). The flap is pulled over medially as far as it will go and sutured. The conjunctiva in the lateral lower fornix is realigned. It is undermined and sutured to the superior edge of the pedicle, re-forming a new canthal angle and somewhat shallower lower fornix. A dehiscence of 11 mm still remains in the lower lid. A full-thickness graft is outlined at the lateral canthus of the ipsilateral upper lid (Fig. 23C).

A full-thickness graft is taken near the lateral canthus of the ipsilateral upper lid, reversed, and sutured into the left lower lid to complete repair of the coloboma (Fig. 23D). The coloboma in the left upper lid is repaired by means of a temporal advancement flap which has been facilitated by the previous cantholysis of the upper arm of the lateral canthal ligament (Fig. 23E) and conjunctival lining of the pedicle.

So much tissue has been lost from the lower lid that it sags after repair (Fig. 23F) and skin from the right upper lid must be used to raise the left lower lid to approximately the same height as the right lower lid (Fig. 23G). The final result is seen in Figure 23H.

Comment: Full-thickness lid grafts are not only feasible but sometimes desirable, since they make possible replacement of large lid loss (more than half a lid) at one sitting thus obviating subsequent surgery.

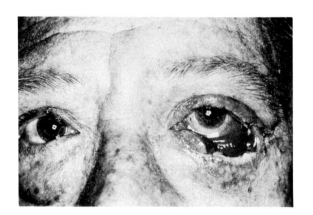

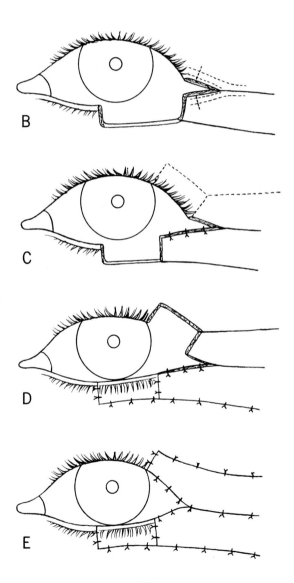

B

C

D

E

36

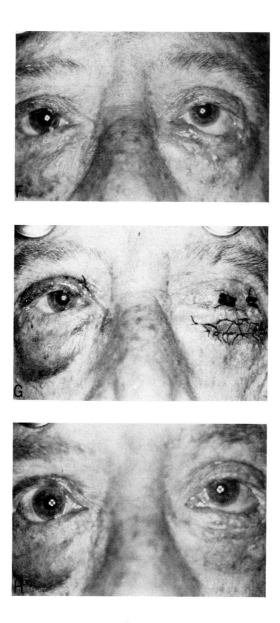

Fig. 23. Full-Thickness Graft Repair for Loss of Over Half a Lid. *A. (opposite page)* Appearance of left lower lid before the repair. *B. (opposite page)* A left lateral canthotomy is made and both arms of the ligament are lysed. A lower lid temporal advancement flap is fashioned. *C. (opposite page)* The lower lid advancement flap is pulled over, lined with mobilized conjunctiva, and sutured. A full-thickness graft and temporal flaps are outlined in the left upper lid. *D. (opposite page)* The full-thickness graft from the left upper lid is reversed and sutured into the left lower lid. A temporal advancement flap is made in the left upper lid. *E. (opposite page)* Repair of the left upper lid is completed. *F.* Result after removal of sutures. *G.* A skin graft from the right upper lid is added to the left lower lid. *H.* Final result.

Healing is remarkably rapid and it is not unusual for the graft to appear normally pink and healthy on the fifth day.

The graft from the donor lid is best taken from the lateral canthal area, where canthotomy, cantholysis, and an advancement graft are available if necessary. Unlike lid skin these full-thickness lid grafts shrink, hence they should be cut generously and transferred immediately to the recipient lid.

Conjunctival lining is rarely a problem in this type of repair. The cut edge of the conjunctiva is dissected up, mobilized, and sutured to the top of the advancement flap when drawn over to create a new lid margin. This makes for a shallower cul-de-sac which is of no consequence with the eye in place. Sometimes buccal mucous membrane must be grafted especially in an anophthalmic socket which must provide ample room for a prosthesis.

Since this type of repair is relatively easy and usually requires only one stage, it may ultimately replace even those technics not requiring sliding grafts for completion. An example is seen in Figure 22.

The two cases just described are prototypes of any transfer of full-thickness lid grafts from one lid to another. Since the tissue loss in many of these cases is great, temporal advancement flaps are added to the free grafts to complete the closure. Thus by combining technics, huge rotated cheek grafts are avoided.

Upper Lid Bridge Flap—Author's Method

PRIMARY INDICATION: *Loss of half or more of lower lid*

Surgical Technic (Fig. 24): The lower lid lesion (Fig. 24A) is resected 4 mm beyond its borders leaving a small nubbin of lid at each canthus. Lateral canthotomy and cantholysis of the lower arm of the canthal ligament are done (Fig. 24B). This permits horizontal approximation of the lid remnants to within 22 mm of each other. By means of two vertical incisions a 22-mm-wide skin advancement flap is fashioned in the lower lid and mobilized (Fig. 24C).

A full-thickness lid advancement flap is fashioned in the ipsilateral upper lid by means of a 24-mm central horizontal incision 4 mm above the lash line and two 15-mm vertical incisions at each end. This flap is split into its component skin-muscle and tarsoconjunctival layers (Fig. 24C).

The tarsoconjunctival layer is pulled down behind the upper lid bridge and sutured to the dissected-up remnant of lower lid conjunctiva with a running suture of 6-0 chromic catgut (Fig. 24D). The upper and lower skin flaps are then united behind the bridge with interrupted sutures of 5-0 silk. The vertical incisions are closed similarly (Fig. 24E and F). About 10 weeks later the upper lid advancement flap is incised below the bridge flap (Fig. 24E, dotted line) and at the sides and allowed to retract.

The advancement flap is sutured to the freshened upper border of the bridge flap and at the sides. The raw edge of the lower lid is sutured, skin-to-conjunctiva, with interrupted sutures of 5-0 silk (Fig. 24G). All sutures are removed on the sixth day. The final result 4 months later is seen in Figure 24H. The upper lid retains complete function, with upward movement (Fig. 24I) and lid closure (Fig. 24J) unimpaired. The cosmetic result is good.

Comment: Study of early ophthalmic literature shows few surgical technics which have not been reported at one time or another. Hence, though no single step in this operation is unique, the combination of technics presented here has never to my knowledge been used for lower lid reconstruction.

The operation consists of (1) the union of upper and lower lid advancement flaps under an upper lid bridge flap; (2) a lateral canthotomy and cantholysis to reduce the *width* of the advancement flaps required; and (3) splitting of the upper advancement flap into layers to increase mobility and to reduce the required *length* of the grafts.

Since the upper lid has much more tissue to spare than the lower, this procedure has a wider use in lower lid reconstruction than the Cutler-Beard (Fig. 31) operation, for instance, in upper lid repairs. A whole lower lid or the greater part of it (as in this case) may be reconstructed by this technic.

Some lesions may extend so far down in the lower lid that an advancement graft will not be enough. In such cases a free skin graft from the contralateral upper lid is simply added to the lower lid at the first operation.

Multiple Advancement Flap—Author's Method

PRIMARY INDICATION: *Loss of more than half of upper lid*

When more than half of the upper lid length is lost, especially laterally, large areas of tissue must be replaced. Several of the commoner methods of repair require the use of tissue from other lids (Figs. 22 through 24). This then entails repair of the donor as well as the recipient lid. However, tissue from other lids may not always be available. Hence any technic which does not go too far afield to borrow tissue from other lids can be exceedingly useful. Such a procedure for upper lid repair without borrowing lower lid tissue is described below.

Surgical Technic (Fig. 25): The lesion involving the outer two-thirds of the left upper lid (Fig. 25A) is resected. This includes three-quarters of lateral lid length. A canthotomy is done and the upper arm of the canthal ligament is severed (Fig. 25B). The upper edge of the

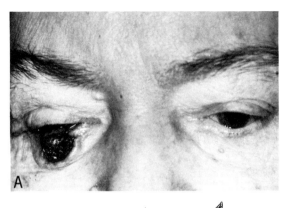

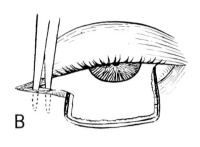

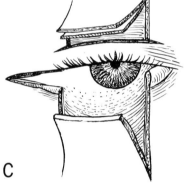

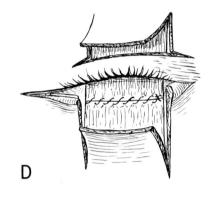

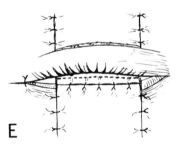

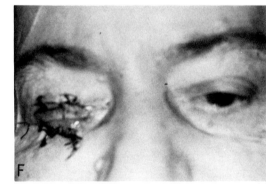

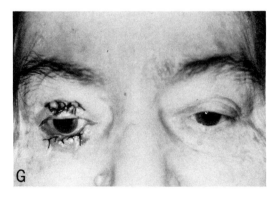

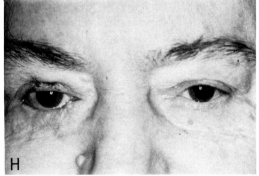

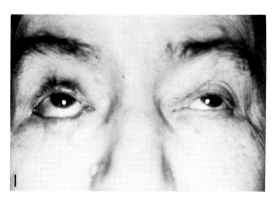
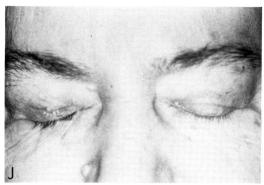

Fig. 24. Lower Lid Reconstruction by Upper Lid Bridge Flap—Author's Technic. A. (*opposite page*) Neoplasm involving most of the right lower lid. B. (*opposite page*) The lesion is resected and lateral canthotomy and cantholysis of lower arm of ligament are done. C. (*opposite page*) A skin advancement flap is fashioned in the lower lid and mobilized. A full-thickness advancement flap is fashioned in the upper lid and split into its two laminae. D. (*opposite page*) The upper lid tarsoconjunctiva is pulled down behind the bridge flap and sutured to the edge of the remaining lower lid conjunctiva. E. (*opposite page*) The upper lid skin-muscle flap is sutured to the lower lid skin flap. F. (*opposite page*) Appearance before suture removal. G. (*opposite page*) The flaps are separated below the bridge flap (dotted line in E). The upper flap is retracted and sutured laterally and to the upper edge of the bridge flap. The raw edge of the lower lid is also sutured skin to conjunctiva. H. (*opposite page*) The final result. I and J. Upper lid movement and lid closure are unimpaired. (From Fox, S. A. *Arch. Ophthalmol.* 85:79, 1971.)

wound is split into skin-muscle and conjunctival layers. The conjunctiva is freely undermined and mobilized by vertical incisions at each end of the split (Fig. 25B, dotted lines). The opposing lower lid margin is also split shallowly enough to give two edges (Fig. 25B) and freshened. The conjunctiva of the upper lid is pulled down and sutured to the tarsoconjunctival edge of the lower lid. A temporal skin flap is outlined at the lateral edge of the wound (Fig. 25C). This is undermined, mobilized, drawn over, and sutured above to the wound margin and below to the skin-muscle lamina of the lower lid. This leaves a central skin dehiscence of about 12 mm. Two vertical skin incisions are made in the lid skin to create a skin flap (Fig. 25D). This is mobilized, drawn down to cover the exposed conjunctiva, and sutured to the lower lid skin-muscle lamina and at the sides (Fig. 25E). The pathology report showed complete extirpation of the lesion.

About 8 weeks later the lids are separated (Fig. 25F). Note that the lid fold is normal and in good position. Opening and closing lid functions are completely unimpaired (Fig. 25G).

Comment: Given an upper lid of an older man which is of normal proportions and has had no previous surgery, it is possible to resect practically the whole lower portion including the full tarsal width and

41

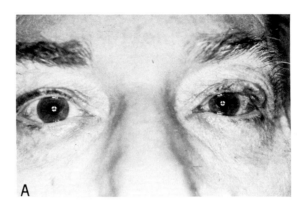

Fig. 25. Upper Lid Reconstruction by Vertical and Horizontal Advancement
Flaps—Author's Technic. A. Neoplasm of the left upper lid. B. The lesion is
resected. Lateral canthotomy and cantholysis of the upper ligament arm are done.
The upper lid wound is split into its laminae and the opposing lower lid is split
(continued)

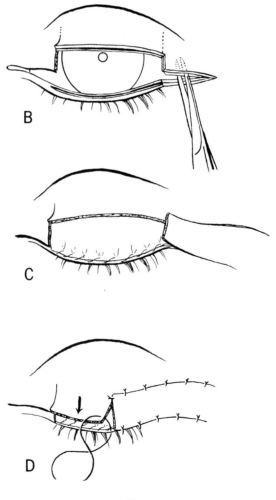

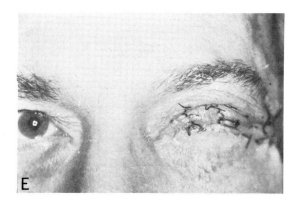

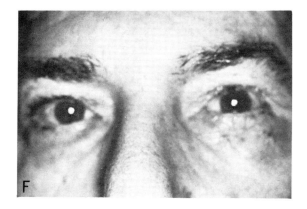

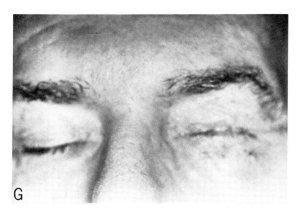

shallowly and freshened. The upper lid conjunctiva is undermined and an advancement flap is made by lateral incisions (dotted lines). *C. (opposite page)* The conjunctival flap is advanced and sutured to the tarsoconjunctival lip of the lower lid. A temporal advancement skin flap is fashioned. *D. (opposite page)* The advancement flap is drawn medially and sutured. Two vertical skin incisions create a vertical advancement flap above. This is drawn down and sutured to the skin-muscle lip of the lower lid. *E.* Appearance before removal of sutures. *F.* Appearance after lid separation. *G.* Lid closure remains unimpaired. (From Fox, S. A. *Arch. Ophthalmol.* to be published.)

then reconstruct the lid by this technic. Upper lids have so much tissue to spare that this can be done without compromising function and still retain a decent cosmetic appearance. Furthermore, the opposing lid has been only minimally involved to the extent of a surgical tarsorrhaphy which heals on opening without residual scar.

Since conjunctiva is elastic and extensible this part of the repair is rarely difficult. Skin replacement is a more formidable problem. It was solved here partly by borrowing temporal skin and partly by using the abundant skin of the lid itself. In lesions of greater width, a simple free skin graft from the opposite lid will work just as well. It was not needed here.

When an upper lid can lose so much of its substance, then contribute additional tissue for its own repair, and still retain normal appearance and function, the interdiction against using upper lid tissue for lower lid repair seems somewhat pointless (see p. 54).

Spontaneous Granulation (Laissez-Faire)—Fox-Beard Method

PRIMARY INDICATION: *Nasocanthal angle lesion of upper and lower lid— separate or combined*

Reconstructions at the medial canthus come close to being the most difficult of all lid repairs. Unfortunately, lesions occur here more frequently, where the nasocanthal angle is narrow and limited by the nose, than at the lateral canthus with its wide-open spaces. In addition, the nasocanthal area houses puncta, canaliculi, canthal ligament, and the lacrimal sac which are often at stake and always in jeopardy unless the lesion is minimal. Preservation of all these important organs is frequently not easy and sometimes not possible.

Early orthodox methods of repair used huge rotated flaps of thick skin from the forehead or nasal region which left ineradicable scars. Free skin grafts are far better but may not be of matching color. Hence the method of laissez-faire, which avoids these pitfalls and still gives a decent result, is a welcome addition to nasocanthal reconstructions. The procedure described below was carried out on a patient who had a basal cell epithelioma of the left nasocanthal angle which had been removed elsewhere several years before but had recurred. The lesion involved the medial ends of both upper and lower lids (Fig. 26A).

Surgical Technic (Fig. 26): The whole nasocanthal mass is removed with a 4-mm margin of normal appearing tissue all around. Dissection includes not only the medial thirds of both lids including the canaliculi, but also the medial canthal ligament and the lacrimal sac.

The lids are everted (Fig. 26B), and the cut conjunctival ends of the upper and lower lids are sutured together with 6-0 chromic catgut to form a new substitute medial fornix (Fig. 26C). The lids are reinverted and a stout double-armed 3-0 silk suture is then passed through the full-thickness cut ends of the lids, taking a good bite. The suture is inserted into the periosteum and the lids drawn over medially (Fig. 26D). A loose petrolated gauze dressing is applied. The wound granulates in rather rapidly as shown in Figure 26E through G, photographs taken 10, 23, and 42 days, respectively, after repair.

The final result is seen in Figure 26H.

Comment: Fastening the lids medially is of paramount importance. Were they not so fastened they would retract laterally and the repair would not be as good. The result is not perfect. The filled-in canthus is usually fuller than its normal counterpart. There is a tendency to cicatricial ptosis due to an occasional shortage of skin; this is easily reparable if desired. Despite these imperfections, the final result is usually as good as and frequently better than that obtained by means of a thick rotated flap or a free skin graft of unmatching color.

Collar-Button Reconstruction—Author's Method

PRIMARY INDICATION: *Lesions involving half or more of upper or lower lid with less marginal or conjunctival than skin involvement*

Basal cell epitheliomas which do not involve the lid margin are usually managed by simple skin resection; sometimes the subjacent muscle is also taken. However, once the margin or margin-cum-conjunctiva has become involved, no matter how little, it is customary to do a full-thickness lid resection of the whole lesion. This has always seemed a waste, since the pathologic report in most cases shows no tarsal involvement. Hence the rationale for the technic described here is based on two observations, clinical and pathologic:

1. Lid epitheliomas, especially the basal cell type, usually start below the lid margin and spread slowly downward and upward to involve the margin and conjunctiva. In a large percentage of these cases the marginal and conjunctival involvement is much less than that of the skin. In a series of 99 cases of basal cell epithelioma 49 showed marginal involvement and 18 also had conjunctival involvement. But in most cases the area of border and conjunctival involvement was considerably less than the area of skin involvement.

2. Serial sections of the lesions showed that most or all of the skin layers were involved. The orbicularis was only rarely involved and then only in old, long-neglected cases. No tarsal invasion was noted in any case, even where the margin and conjunctiva were invaded. One would expect the meibomian gland openings to facilitate tarsal invasion by marginal neoplasms, but they do not, as repeated pathologic studies have shown. This is not to say that tarsal invasion never occurs. It probably does; but rarely.

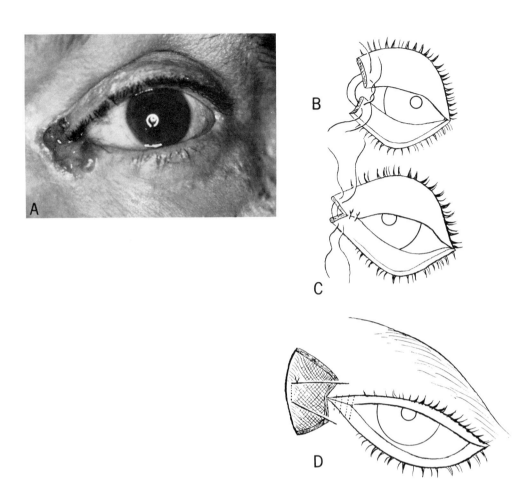

Fig. 26.   Repair by Spontaneous Granulation (Laissez-Faire)—Fox-Beard Method. A. Left nasocanthal neoplasm.   B. and C. After resection of the lesion and involved portions of the lids, a new substitute medial fornix is created.   D. The remaining lid portions are pulled over and sutured to the nasal periosteum. E, F, and G. (*opposite page*) Appearance of granulating wound 10, 23, and 42 days later.   H. (*opposite page*) Final result.

Surgical Technic (Fig. 27):   Starting at the lid margin an incision is made through skin and muscle all around the skin lesion including 4 mm of healthy tissue. Then starting at the margin again, 4 mm to each side of the involved marginal (and conjunctival, if involved) area, two vertical incisions are made downward through tarsoconjunctiva. These incisions are curved in to meet each other below the tarsus in healthy conjunctiva. The ends of the skin-muscle and tarsoconjunctival incisions at the border are united by incisions through the gray line. The tissue thus outlined containing the whole lesion—the larger skin lesion and lesser tarsoconjunctival lesion—is split away from the rest of the lid en bloc.

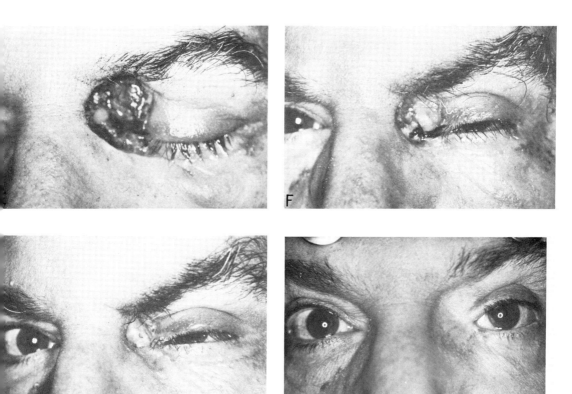

Since the amount of skin-muscle resected is always much more than tarsoconjunctiva, the resected portion resembles an old-fashioned collar-button (Fig. 27, *inset*)— hence the name. Many variations of this technic are possible. A few are described below:

1. A medium-sized lesion involving the center of the lid can be corrected by horizontal tarsoconjunctival closure and vertical skin-muscle flap. In such a case a collar-button resection is done (Fig. 28). With the help of canthotomy and cantholysis (if necessary) the tarsoconjunctival wound

Fig. 27. Collar-Button Method of Lid Reconstruction— Arthur's Technic. Schema of resection. The anterior larger resection is of skin-muscle lamina. The posterior lesser resection is tarsoconjunctival. *Inset* shows collar-button shape of excised tissue. (From Fox, S. A. *Arch. Ophthalmol.* 65:345-352, 1961.

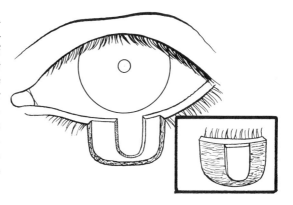

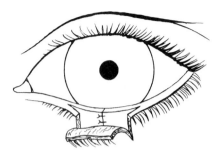

Fig. 28. Collar-Button Method of Lid Reconstruction: Medium-Sized Central Lesion—Author's Technic. Resection of lesion and repair by horizontal tarsoconjunctival closure and vertical skin flap.

is closed in the usual fashion. If the tumor is shallow, it is possible to fashion a vertical sliding skin flap, which is drawn up and sutured to the lid margin as shown.

2. A medium-sized lesion at the lateral canthus can be managed by another variation of this technic. Here repair is attained by means of horizontal closure of the tarsoconjunctival wound as in the previous case. But the skin-muscle wound is closed by a temporal sliding flap, thus taking advantage of the lesion's position. After collar-button resection of the lesion, canthotomy and cantholysis are done and a temporal sliding flap is fashioned (Fig. 29A). The tarsoconjunctival wound is closed and the temporal flap is pulled over the bared tarsus and sutured (Fig. 29B).

3. Finally, when the lesion is large, repair may be attained by a free whole-skin graft. The lesion is resected collar-button fashion and lateral canthotomy and cantholysis are done (Fig. 30A). The tarsoconjunctival wound is closed as in the two previous cases. A free graft is taken from the ipsilateral upper lid and used to cover the lower lid dehiscence (Fig. 30B). The upper margin of the graft is sutured to the opposing lid margin, which has been freshened.

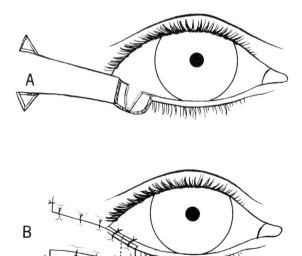

Fig. 29. Collar-Button Method of Lid Reconstruction: Lateral Lesion —Author's Technic. *A.* The canthal lesion is resected collar-button fashion, and a lateral advancement flap is fashioned. Note Burow's triangles to counteract wrinkling. *B.* The tarsoconjunctiva is sutured and the temporal skin flap is advanced medially to close the wound.

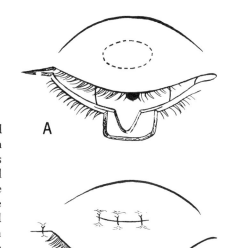

Fig. 30. Collar-Button Method of Lid Reconstruction: Large Central Lesion —Author's Technic. A. The lesion is resected collar-button fashion and lateral canthotomy and cantholysis of the lower arm of the canthal ligament are done. B. The tarsoconjunctiva is closed horizontally. A free-skin graft is taken from the ipsilateral upper lid to close the wound in the lower lid. The upper lip of the graft is sutured to the freshened margin of the upper lid.

Comment: It is important to make sure that the neoplasm has been completely excised. This can be achieved by removing sufficient healthy tissue all around, as described previously, and confirming the results by means of frozen section examination. Canthotomy or canthotomy-cum-cantholysis is usually done. This always facilitates tarsoconjunctival wound closure.

In summary, the collar-button technic is suggested for (1) epitheliomas of the lid which (2) involve the lid margin or margin-cum-conjunctiva and in which (3) the involvement of the skin is much greater than that of the margin (and conjunctiva).

Wheeler pointed out long ago that the tarsus is a low-grade tissue which heals poorly. Perhaps this also accounts for its failure to be invaded by neoplasms. But, however the case, replacement of this inelastic, relatively avascular tissue is not always easily accomplished. Any procedure, therefore, which minimizes tarsal loss facilitates lid repair. The collar-button technic considerably reduces the amount of tarsal resection and often permits closure of the tarsoconjunctival wound directly, obviating the tarsal grafting which might be necessary if the old technics were used.

Lower Lid Bridge Flap—Cutler-Beard Method (Modified)

PRIMARY INDICATION: *Loss of half or less of upper lid*

This procedure was reported some 15 years ago and is still a useful technic for reconstruction of less than half an upper lid.

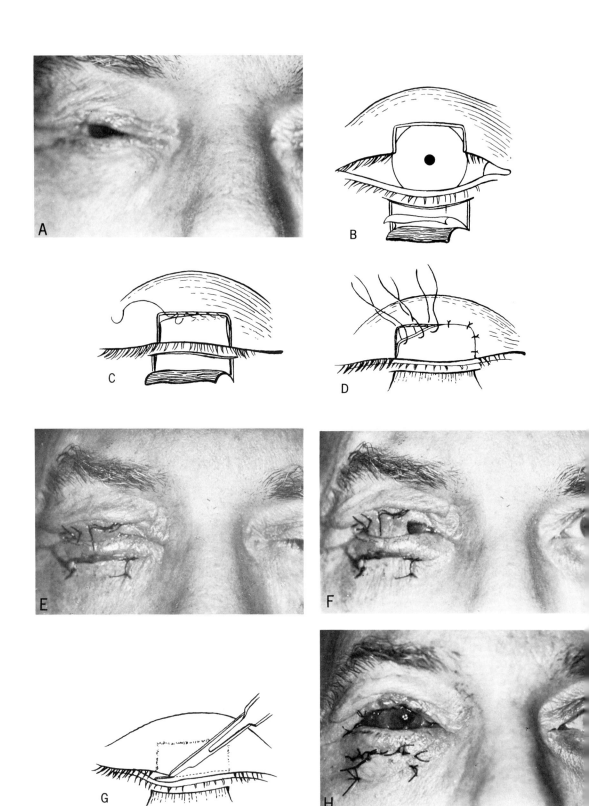

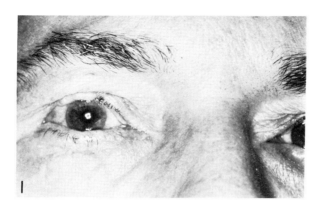

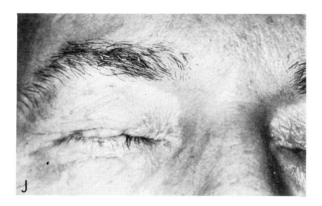

Fig. 31. Lower Lid Bridge Flap Technic for Upper Lid Reconstruction—Cutler-Beard Method (Modified).   *A. (opposite page)* Coloboma of the right upper lid. *B. (opposite page)* The margins of the upper lid coloboma are freshened and the wound made rectangular. A full-thickness advancement flap is fashioned in the lower lid and split into layers. *C. (opposite page)* The conjunctiva is drawn up and sutured to the posterior edge of the coloboma.   *D and E. (opposite page)* The skin is drawn up and sutured.   *F. (opposite page)* Note the free play given the lower lid flap as the upper lid moves up.   *G. (opposite page)* After 8 weeks the lids are separated.   *H. (opposite page)* The upper lid edge is sutured and the lower lid flap retracted and sutured back into position.   *I.* Result after suture removal.   *J.* Closure is complete.

Surgical Technic (Fig. 31):   The upper lid defect (Fig. 31A) is prepared by freshening the borders and shaping them as closely as possible to a rectangle in order to facilitate repair. A full-thickness lower lid horizontal incision is made just below the attached tarsal border to match the upper lid dehiscence. Two full-thickness vertical incisions are then made from each end of this incision downward to create a rectangular advancement flap. The flap is split into its two component layers (Fig. 31B). The conjunctival layer is drawn up behind the bridge flap and sutured to the posterior edge of the upper lid coloboma with 6-0 chromic sutures (Fig. 31C). The skin-muscle flap is then drawn up and sutured to the coloboma skin edges with interrupted sutures of 5-0 silk (Fig. 31D and E). The lower border of the bridge flap is *not* sutured to the advancement flap (Fig. 31F).

The wound is covered with a nonadhesive firm supportive dressing without pressure. The eye is dressed in 5 days and loose sutures removed. All sutures are removed 1 or 2 days later.

After 7 or 8 weeks, the new upper lid margin is marked out on the upper lid with antiseptic dye by a line slightly convex downward to counteract possible retraction. The lids are divided (Fig. 31G) and the raw upper lid edge is sutured, skin-to-conjunctiva, with interrupted sutures of 6-0 silk. The lower lid flap is freed at the sides so it can resume its position in the lower lid. It is then sutured to the freshened lower edge of the bridge flap and at the sides in layers (Fig. 31H). Sutures are removed 5 to 7 days later and the final result is seen in Figure 31I. Closure is unimpeded (Fig. 31J).

Comment: There are two modifications of the original technic which I consider important: (1) splitting the advancement flap gives greater mobility and elasticity to the tissues and allows a wider repair; (2) since the advancement flap is not sutured to the bridge flap, it moves freely with the movement of the upper lid (Fig. 31F). This free play keeps it from contracting and forestalls a later tendency to ectropion due to lower lid shortening.

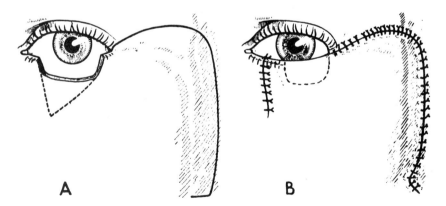

A   **B**

Fig. 32. Rotated Cheek Flap for Lower Lid Reconstruction—Mustardé's Technic. A. Resection of lesion and triangle below the lid. Rotated cheek flap is outlined, and canthotomy and lower arm cantholysis are done. B. The cheek flap is rotated over and the wounds are closed. If necessary the flap is lined with nasal or buccal mucous membrane. (From Mustardé, J. C. *Repair and Reconstruction in the Orbital Region.* Baltimore, Williams & Wilkins, 1966.)

Little tension is exerted on the flap sutures. In most cases there is adequate lower fornix tissue to provide for an upper lid defect of reasonable size. However, this type of repair is best accomplished if the upper lid coloboma is not too wide. Notching of the upper lid may occur and is repaired in the usual way. Scar retraction and ectropion in the lower lid sometimes have to be corrected at a later date. Trichiasis has been noted and is best repaired by a tarsoconjunctival graft (Fig. 56).

A complication which is rarely mentioned but which may occur is fusion of the raw edge of the bridge flap to the intact lower lid skin during the healing process. Surprisingly, this can happen even though the pedicle flap is mobile and not sutured to the lower lid. Adhesion may be prevented by frequent separation of the hammock flap from the lower lid by inserting a glass rod and running it from one end to the other. If healing does occur, the skin adhesions must be dissected away and the skin wound in the lower lid closed separately. This is another reason for not suturing the raw edge of the bridge flap to the lid.

Rotated Cheek Flap—Mustardé's Method

PRIMARY INDICATION: *Loss of half or more of lower lid*
Recently there has been a minor revival of the giant rotated cheek flap for lower lid reconstruction.

Surgical Technic (Fig. 32): The lesion is resected triangularly with a 4-mm margin of healthy lid tissue on each side. The downward incisions must be quite long to permit mobilization and rotation of the cheek flap medially. The flap of cheek skin is incised as outlined (Fig. 32A). Canthotomy and cantholysis of the lower arm of the canthal ligament are done to improve mobility, and the flap is rotated medially and sutured. If conjunctival replacement is needed, buccal or nasal mucosa may be used (Fig. 32B).

If normal lid tissue can be saved, it is sutured to the flap in layers. The medial and lateral cheek wounds are closed using subcuticular sutures if necessary. To prevent lateral sagging later, the heavy cheek flap must be sutured high up where it crosses the orbital rim. A pressure bandage is applied for 48 hours and sutures are removed on the sixth day.

Comment: There is no doubt that a lower lid can be reconstructed in this way. But the objection is not only to the scars below the lid and at the side of the face but to the character of the lid itself. It is often heavier and more lifeless looking than a lid constructed by other procedures described above.

The reason given for reversion to large, primitive rotated pedicles is that use of upper lid tissue for lower lid repair is detrimental to the upper lid, both functionally and cosmetically. After a surgical lifetime of successfully using upper lid tissue for lower lid repair without incurring cosmetic or functional harm to the upper lid, I can but disagree—emphatically. The most cursory glance at the repairs depicted in this chapter will show that these procedures do not damage the upper lid.

Addendum

The past 10 or 15 years have seen a deepening of interest in ophthalmic plastic surgery which has paralled a quickening and growth in the whole fabric of this somewhat esoteric ophthalmic subspecialty. The changes are obvious: Classic lid splitting and lid halving are moribund; newer, simpler, and more daring technics are replacing them. The procedures described above are links in the gradual evolution of technics suitable to the specialized requirements of lid surgery.

However, not all changes are advances. Occasional retreats are caught up in this new climate of forward progress, and old procedures are rediscovered, refurbished, and reported as new. An example is the recent exhumation of the king-sized rotated cheek flap with its princely scars, described above. Although the procedure itself is Middle Aged, the excuses for its disinterment are the hobgoblin that borrowing upper lid tissue for lower lid repair, however slight, is lethal to upper lid well-being, and (2) that the lower lid is really not necessary and absence of part or all of it can be tolerated despite discomfort from conjunctival exposure and tearing. (The strength of the latter argument is immediately compromised by the fact that the recommended procedure involves a generously proportioned rotated cheek flap to reconstruct the "unnecessary" lower lid.)

I have chosen this particular example because I consider it among those constituting a backward step in time and a backward leap in technic. According to this new surgical ethic, some of the technics described above should not have been used and, having been used, should not have provided the victims with good-looking, well-functioning lids.

It is frightening, after many years of satisfactorily and successfully using upper lid tissue for lower lid repair, to discover that the upper lid is so delicate and vulnerable that loss of even a modicum of its tissue will endanger its functional and cosmetic integrity. Apparently only intervention from on high has saved unwary surgeons and their hapless patients from disaster. It is as if the progress begun with Reverdin and carried down to the present day had been completely forgotten.

And Tagliacozzi rides again!

The interdiction against using upper lid tissue for lower lid repair after all these years is not easy to understand. It is conceivable that upper lid tissue might for some reason be unavailable, that the patient himself might object to having surgical liberties taken with his normal lid, or that some unusual circumstance might make the rotated cheek flap no more undesirable than any other technic. I can even understand—almost—a surgeon cleaving to this one technic and abandoning all others. What is hard to understand is the edict that "there cannot be any justification for utilizing . . . the upper lid to reconstruct the . . . lower lid."

Are all the successful repairs which broke this rule for many years pure happenstance? Or are there several ways of achieving good lower lid repairs, one of which is using upper lid tissue? When an upper lid can lose much of its substance and still retain normal function and appearance, as shown above, the case against using upper lid tissue for lower lid repair becomes untenable.

REFERENCES

Ballen, P. H. Reconstruction of lower eyelid with upper lid composite graft. *Ophthalmol. Surg.* 1:31-37, 1970.

Callahan, A. A free composite lid graft. *Arch. Ophthalmol.* 45:539, 1951.

Cutler, N. L., and Beard, C. Reconstruction of upper lid. *Am. J. Ophthalmol.* 39:1, 1955.

Fox, S. A. Lid halving with variations. *Arch. Ophthalmol.* 65:672, 1961.

Fox, S. A. Autogenous free full-thickness grafts. *Am. J. Ophthalmol.* 67:941, 1969.

Fox, S. A. A procedure for lower lid reconstruction. *Arch. Ophthalmol.* 85:79, 1971.

Fox, S. A., and Beard, C. Spontaneous lid repair. *Am. J. Ophthalmol.* 58:947, 1964.

Lawson, G. On the successful transplantation of portions of skin for the closure of large granulating surfaces. *Lancet* 2:708, 1870.

Le Fort, L. C. Blépharoplastie par un lambeau complétement detaché du bras et reporté à la face. *Bull. Mem. Soc. Chir. Paris* 1:39, 1872.

Mustardé, J. C. *Repair and Reconstruction in the Orbital Region.* Baltimore, Williams & Wilkins, 1966.

Ollier, L. Des greffes cutanees. *C. R. Acad. Sci.* 74:817, 1872.

Reverdin, J. L. Greffe épidermique: Experience faite dans le service de M. le Docteur Guyon à l'hôpital Necker. *Gaz. Hop.* 43:15, 1870.

Sichel, A. Blépharoplastie par greffe dermique. *Bull. Acad. Med.* 4:574, 1875.

Thiersch, C. Über die feineren anatomischer Veranderungen bei Augenheilung von des Haut auf Granulationen. *Arch. Klin. Chir.* 17:318, 1874.

Wolfe, J. R. A new method for performing plastic operations. *Med. Times Gaz.* 1:608, 1876.

Youens, M. T., Westphal, C., Bartfield, F. T. Jr., and Youens, H. T. Jr. Full-thickness lower lid transplant. *Arch. Ophthalmol.* 77:226, 1967.

CHAPTER 4

Ptosis

NEW ETIOLOGIC CLASSIFICATION

Blepharoptosis is *sui generis*. In most common lid affections it is the acquired, not the congenital, cases that are seen most frequently and are most important—for example, neoplasms, entropion, and ectropion. But ptosis, the lid anomaly most often seen by the ophthalmologist, is congenital in more than half of the affected patients. This division of ptosis into two main types has remained unchanged since Bowman reported his first levator resection.

On the face of it, nothing seems simpler or less obscure than a classification which divides ptosis cases clinically into congenital cases present at birth and acquired cases which appear sometime after birth. But dogmatic custom and unquestioning habit often prolong and protect old, sometimes revered, usages long after they have become inadequate. This, I am afraid, has happened to our old clinical classification of ptosis. We have stubbornly clung to this arrangement in the face of substantial etiologic questions and new contradictory facts (especially concerning the acquired ptoses), which have plagued us and which still remain unanswered.

The inadequacy of the old classification became acutely apparent to me when I reviewed my last 200 ptosis cases. I divided the cases into the hitherto accepted two main groups: congenital and acquired. I found that 147 (73.5 per cent) were present at birth and hence classed as congenital and 53 (26.5 per cent) were in the acquired category since they appeared after—sometimes long after—birth.

Congenital Ptosis

Of the congenital cases about three-quarters were unilateral and one-quarter bilateral; on further subdivision they fell into easily assorted groups as follows:

Simple	91	(45.5%)
Complicated		
By other lid anomalies	23	(11.5%)
By ophthalmoplegias	20	(10.0%)
Synkinetic	13	(6.5%)

Of the simple cases three-quarters were unilateral and one-quarter bilateral. The complicated cases were associated with ophthalmoplegias and/or other lid anomalies. The ophthalmoplegias most commonly but not always included superior rectus weakness due to the common anlage with the levator.

The synkinetic cases were mostly the Marcus Gunn type of paradoxic (and complicated) ptoses with their still unsolved enigmatic etiology which often compound our confusion by disappearing inexplicably as the patient grows older. This was pointed out by Robert Marcus Gunn himself when he originally described the pterygoid-levator synkinesis in 1883. We know little more about this curious clinical abnormality now than we did then. It seems due to misdirection of Nn III and VII. But how explain the gradual improvement and loss of jaw-winking which undoubtedly occurs with aging? Is there a readjustment of the innervating fibers or does the misdirection come undone? Both explanations are hard to believe and harder to explain. Since paradoxic means "opposed to common sense," this disorder is well named. However, there is no uncertainty about the fact of its presence at birth. It is not inherited; hence congenital it is.

But what about the 23 patients with ptosis complicated by other lid anomalies? Of these, 8 had rare lid malformations such as coloboma, ectropion, entropion, and epiblepharon. But 15 presented the so-called mongoloid syndrome—bilateral ptosis, phimosis, epicanthus, and (more rarely) telecanthus. For some time now we have known that these are inherited characteristics, although no chromosomal aberrations have yet been found.

Actually mongoloid stigmata are part of Waardenburg's embryonic fixation syndrome, which may also include the much rarer hypoplasia of the caruncle, peripheral muscle dysplasias, and other uncommon anomalies. All these can be independently inherited, but those most often seen by the ophthalmologist are bilateral ptosis, phimosis, epicanthus, and (less commonly) telecanthus. The hereditary pattern is an autosomal dominant occurring equally in and transmitted equally through both sexes. Thus while the syndrome's name is not an apt description of its most common features, the condition is obviously neither a nameless orphan nor a changeling as has been stated. Hence in these 15 patients the ptosis, present at birth, was

transmitted before gestation and therefore, being heredo-familial, was or-
dained before birth and therefore not congenital as we understand the
word. And our smooth waters of classification are becoming somewhat roiled.

Thus, instead of 147 (73.5 per cent) cases of congenital ptosis, we have
only 132 (66 per cent) cases which, simple or complicated, were present at
birth but were not inherited and are therefore congenital.

Acquired Ptosis

The 53 (26.5 per cent) acquired cases are classified as follows:

Neurogenic	3	(1.5%)
Traumatic	13	(6.5%)
Senile	17	(8.5%)
Myogenic	20	(10.0%)

Obviously the neurogenic and traumatic cases are of a different order
from the other types of acquired ptosis. Not only are they absent at birth,
but they are always due to known and ascertainable causes which occur
after birth. They are truly acquired.

The etiology of senile ptosis is cloudier. We attribute senile ptosis
to the generalized muscular atonicity which accompanies aging and which,
we presume, includes the levators. Since this type of ptosis first manifests
itself in the older generation, it is called senile and would seem to be
acquired. Yet frequently the levators are the only atonic muscles in these
patients and one wonders why only the levators and no other muscles have
aged. But in the present stage of our knowledge we have to classify senile
ptosis as acquired, although we are not always sure why or how.

The late-appearing myogenic ptoses fall into three distinct divisions:

Heredofamilial (bilateral)	13	(6.5%)
Nonfamilial (unilateral)	5	(2.5%)
Myasthenia gravis	2	(1.0%)

Of the 13 cases of familial ptosis, 2 belonged in the group of primary
muscular atrophy described by Duke-Elder (see below). I have called the
other 11 "progressive familial myopathic ptosis." In all these patients the
lids appeared normal at birth but began to show signs of ptosis later in life
anywhere from the second to the fifth or sixth decade. Since 85 per cent
described a similar disorder in other members of the family, the process
is undoubtedly heredofamilial. In addition, every patient with familial ptosis
had involvement of one, some, or all the other extraocular muscles. No
other musculature in the body was involved.

How classify these cases? Obviously they are not in the same category as the traumatic or neurogenic ptosis whose postnatal acquired etiology

is unquestioned. Although hitherto classed as acquired, the familial ptoses were acquired only in the sense that the malfunction appeared after birth. They occur after birth, but are they acquired after birth as we understand the term "acquired?" Like the mongoloid syndrome, they have sprouted from seeds planted before birth. Hence these 13 cases are not acquired but inherited, and reduce our total of acquired cases from 53 (26.5 per cent) to 40 (20.0 per cent). The need for a modification of our classification appears even more strong.

The 2 cases of myasthenia gravis are obviously acquired and need no further discussion.

I have classified the remaining 5 cases as "late spontaneous unilateral ptosis." They appeared as follows:

SEX	AGE OF ONSET	EYE
Female	48 Years	OS
Female	27 Years	OS
Female	20 Years	OD
Male	11 Years	OS
Male	9 Years	OS

These are perhaps the most inexplicable of all the cases in this report (with the possible exception of the Marcus Gunn genre). They are not common but undoubtedly every ophthalmologist has seen one or two such cases and has tried to figure out their etiology, as I have, with something less than complete success. No history of other familial involvement was obtained from any of the patients in this series. In all, the spontaneous appearance of ptosis long after birth was proved by serial photographs and unimpeachable investigated histories.

Histologic examination showed the same nonspecific levator dystrophy as is found in the congenital ptoses. No other extraocular muscles were involved.

This type of ptosis should not be confused with the intermittent levator weakness seen in infants and young children when they are tired or sick and which becomes more obvious as the years accumulate. Such levator weakness makes itself known shortly after birth and is obviously of congenital origin. In the 5 cases described here, there was no sign of levator weakness at birth or for years thereafter. But something caused these lids to droop, although no other pathology was found after complete physical and neurologic investigation. These ptoses are acquired; but why and how? Idiopathic is an overworked adjective, but no other seems to fit here.

We cannot indulge here in wide philosophic speculation on etiology. But briefly, it should be of interest to ophthalmologists that the more we delve into this interesting and somewhat mysterious group of familial myogenic ptoses, the more involved classification becomes. For the whole group is itself susceptible to division into a number of subgroups, of which three have been cited by Duke-Elder:

1. Primary muscular atrophy (late familial ptosis), in which the ptosis is usually the only symptom
2. Dystrophia myotonica, in which there are dystrophies not only of the extraocular musculature but also of the face, neck, and extremities
3. Myasthenia gravis, a nonfamilial acquired ptosis

Recently other subgroups have been added:

4. The congenital [sic] fibrosis syndrome (extensively described by Laughlin), characterized by bilateral ptosis and gradual fibrosis of all the extraocular muscles
5. Oculopharyngeal muscular dystrophy (described by Victor *et al.*), characterized by dysphagia and progressive bilateral ptosis

To these we may add the two other subgroups described in this chapter:

6. Progressive familial myopathic ptosis, characterized by bilateral ptosis and involvement of one, some, or all of the extraocular (and no other) muscles of one or both eyes
7. Late spontaneous unilateral ptosis

Of these seven groups, myasthenia gravis, although myogenic, is obviously acquired, and late spontaneous unilateral ptosis will also have to be classed as acquired until we learn different or better. The other five groups are all inherited.

It may well be that these five inherited subgroups—they are neither congenital nor acquired—are not individual clinical subdivisions and that the attempt to isolate them into autonomous entities is useless and, indeed, impossible. However, each one contains a distinctly typical pathologic core around which similar appearing cases may be grouped. If the peripheries of these subgroups merge, it only proves that human pathology does not always lend itself to precise classification or that we are not yet wise enough to perceive the difference. Other subgroups will doubtless be added in the future.

Obviously the etiology and classification of the ptoses is far from settled. We know a great deal more about the subject than in the days of Bowman. But there are areas about which we know no more—or as little— as was known 100 years ago, and by now our old clinical classification begins to look somewhat battered. Obviously the deeper we delve into the etiologies of these cases, the more vague they become until they fade into almost complete obscurity. The very fact that new groups keep popping up shows that their classification into nice cohesive entities is far from settled.

From what has been said above, the following etiologic classification of the ptoses would seem to be a truer reflection of the known facts and ignorances than the old clinical grouping to which we have paid obeisance for so many years:

Congenital
   Simple
   Complicated
         By ophthalmoplegias
         By other lid anomalies
         Synkinetic (paradoxic)

Acquired
   Senile
   Traumatic
   Late spontaneous
   Neurogenic (Horner's syndrome, etc.)
   Myogenic (myasthenia gravis, etc.)

Heredofamilial
   At birth
   Embryonic Fixation (Mongoloid) syndrome
   Late appearing
         Various myogenic subgroups

My aim has been not to tear down old classifications which have served us well for so long, but to amend and modernize in the light of what we have learned from genetics and chromosomal studies during recent years. I do not propose the above classification as anything but a basis for discussion. Much still remains to be learned. For instance, the new subclass heredofamilial comprises both congenital and acquired ptoses and is certainly sufficiently different in manifestation to warrant a grouping of its own. On the other hand, we have no unequivocal etiologic answer to the bilateral senile and the unilateral late spontaneous ptoses here reported. The inherited myogenic ptoses are fractionated into several groups which may or may not deserve independence. This classification is not—cannot be—final. Facts come, uncertainties go, classifications change.

Pseudoptosis

Pseudoptosis has not been discussed here because there is little new to say about it. It includes all drooping of the lid not due to levator weakness—a lid displaced downward by edema, by tumor, by cicatri, or by absence, retroplacement, or shrinkage of the globe; senile lid atrophy; and blepharochalasis. A form of pseudoptosis due to superior rectus weakness should not be forgotten. The ptosis may be due to the patient's effort to block out a diplopia brought on by this muscular weakness. The condition can be alleviated by repair of the offending extraocular muscles; levator surgery is not indicated.

SURGERY OF PTOSIS

Although the etiology of ptosis is far from settled, surgical treatment of ptosis seems so set today that it suffers from the doldrums. Little has been produced currently which should shake us from our technics of the past 10 years.

Further study from a surgical viewpoint of the 200 cases discussed above shows the following:

TYPE OF OPERATION	TOTAL	CONGENITAL	ACQUIRED
Levator resection	59%	52%	88%
Frontalis suspension	41%	48%	12%

Although levator resection accounted for almost 60 per cent of all operations, the congenital cases were about evenly divided in the kind of repair done. In the acquired cases, however, levator resection was by far the most common operation because patients with senile, traumatic, myogenic, and even neurogenic ptoses all have a modicum of levator action which favors levator resection. Also these types of ptoses usually occur in patients old enough to cooperate in thorough study and identification of small amounts of levator action.

The choice of the type of surgery as well as the need for preoperative study have been extensively discussed in the literature and need no elaboration here. It suffices to say that I prefer levator resection for all ptosis patients with at least 2 mm of levator action. With less levator action, frontalis suspension with autogenous fascia or skin is the technic of choice (see below).

It is not always easy to detect small amounts of levator action, especially in the uncooperative young. It might therefore be wise to postpone surgery until time and sufficient examination have furnished enough evidence to warrant a choice of operative procedure.

The question whether ptosis is due to sympathetic or parasympathetic causes is occasionally broached as a factor in the choice of surgery. The distinction may be based on pupillary size, with the sympathetic ptosis having a smaller pupil. However, this is a rather unsatisfactory test because pupillary size does not change often enough or appreciably enough to make a diagnosis always possible. The cocaine test is more reliable: There is no dilation in the sympathetic type of ptosis. Kestenbaum has pointed out that the lower lid of the ptotic eye is usually higher than the lower lid of the normal eye. To me the whole question is somewhat academic because I have never seen a ptosis of any degree which can be repaired by surgery on Müller's (sympathetic) muscle alone.

The only new tendency—if it may be called new—is to do less and less surgery on the horns in levator resection because cutting the horns increases the ptosis and tends to diminish the effect of levator shortening.

Of course, in the larger corrections horns must be cut, but in the presence of an appreciable levator action (8 mm or more) the horns should be cut minimally or not at all.

I prefer the anterior approach to the levator with the amount of levator resection directly dependent on the amount of *levator action* and not on the amount of ptosis. For the apparent amount of ptosis may bear no relation to the action of the levator. It is possible to have what appears to be a small amount of congenital ptosis with relatively little levator action. On the other hand, traumatic ptosis may be almost total and yet be associated with good levator action.

Levator Resection

LEVATOR RESECTION BY THE ANTERIOR ROUTE

I prefer to use local anesthesia whenever possible. It is sometimes helpful in swelling the bulk of the thinned atrophic tissues of older patients. The exceptions are, of course, when the patient is too young (or too old) to cooperate. Some adults insist on general anesthesia and must be accommodated.

Surgical Technic (Fig. 33): An incision is made through skin and muscle about 1 mm below the upper tarsal border and the skin-muscle lamina is dissected downward; care must be taken not to go too far down into the area of the cilia roots. The dissection is then carried upward sufficiently high to uncover an adequate amount of levator. The orbital fascia and subjacent fat are thus exposed and the junction of union between fascia and levator is identified and freed (Fig. 33A). When this is done orbital fat sometimes presents and should be resected without hesitation.

The levator aponeurosis is buttonholed at one end of the upper tarsal border, blunt-pointed scissors inserted, and the undermining carried across to the other end, separating it and Müller's muscle from the subjacent conjunctiva. Thus the conjunctiva remains intact and need not be sutured later. A ptosis clamp is inserted into the undermined area between levator and conjunctiva and locked. The levator (cum Müller's) is now cut from its attachment to the upper tarsal border (Fig. 33B).

The levator is raised and freed from the underlying conjunctiva by careful dissection (Fig. 33C). If the conjunctiva is buttonholed (as it sometimes is) the cut, if large, should be closed with 6-0 plain catgut sutures which absorb readily and hence cause least possible irritation to the cornea.

If levator action is only moderate or slight (up to 7 or 8 mm) the horns of the levator aponeurosis are cut to free it (Fig. 33D). However, where levator action is not seriously reduced (as in traumatic ptosis or in Horner's syndrome), the horns are not cut.

Three double-armed 4-0 chromic sutures (5-0 chromic in the very young) are inserted—equally spaced—in the tarsus about 3 or 4 mm from

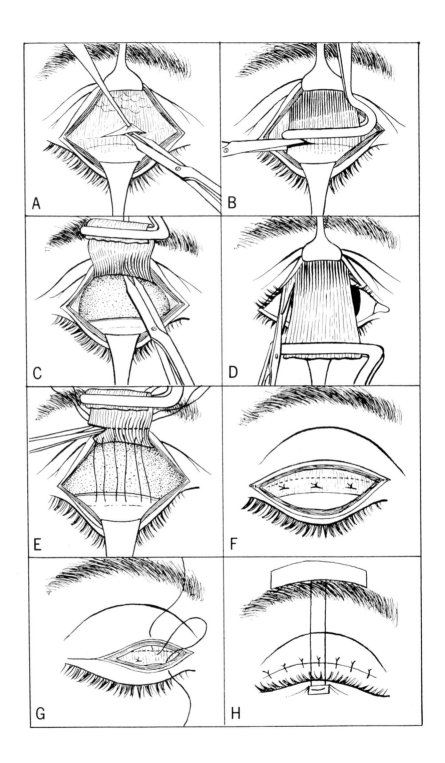

Fig. 33. Levator Resection by External Approach—Author's Technic. *A.* The skin-muscle lamina is incised about 1 mm below the upper tarsal border and undermined upward and downward. The exposed orbital fascia is dissected away from the levator. *B.* Levator and Müller's muscles are undermined at the upper tarsal border. A ptosis clamp is inserted and the tissues cut from their attachment. *C.* Levator and Müller's muscles are undermined upward. Note the conjunctiva is *not* cut. *D.* The horns are cut if necessary. *E.* Three equally spaced double-armed chromic sutures are inserted in the tarsus, then into the levator from behind forward. The excess levator is resected. *F.* The sutures are tied and the levator thus pulled down into the tarsus. *G.* The skin is closed. See text for method of lid fold formation. *H.* A modified Frost suture pulls the lower lid up over the cornea. (From Fox, S. A. *Ophthalmic Plastic Surgery,* ed. 4. New York, Grune & Stratton, 1970.)

the upper border. If more lifting power is needed they are inserted a couple of millimeters lower down. They are then carried up and passed through the levator from behind forward as far from the cut end as is required by the degree of ptosis. The excess levator is then resected (Fig. 33E). The sutures are tied and the levator is thus brought down onto the surface of the tarsus (Fig. 33F).

The skin-muscle incision is closed as follows: Four equally spaced 5-0 silk sutures are passed through the lower lip of the wound, through the upper tarsal border, then through the upper lip of the wound (Fig. 33G). This creates a good lid fold without the need for special sutures. Additional skin sutures are added for good closure. In the young, 5-0 plain catgut is used to close the wound so that sutures need not be removed. A modified Frost suture is inserted and the lower lid pulled up over the cornea (Fig. 33H). The Frost suture is removed on the second or third day because in the usual case the upper lid is heavy and edematous at this time and covers the cornea without any help from the lower lid.

Comment: One of the advantages of an anterior approach to the levator is that the conjunctiva need not be cut and then sutured, as is seen in this technic. This spares the patient the discomfort caused by the sutures rubbing against the cornea. At worst they could cause a good deal of corneal damage.

LEVATOR RESECTION BY THE POSTERIOR ROUTE

Levator resection by the conjunctival route is often used as a secondary procedure and in those cases of lesser ptosis and better levator action in which complete exposure of the levator is not of critical importance. In these circumstances the Iliff and the modified Blaskovics procedures are useful. These have been widely reported in the literature and need no repetition here.

COMMON COMPLICATIONS OF LEVATOR RESECTION

It has been stated that cicatricial entropion of the upper lid may develop due to conjunctival loss if more than one levator resection operation is done by the posterior route. This is contrary to my experience. Entropion is caused more commonly by too much levator resection than by conjunctival loss. The levator constitutes part of the posterior lid lamina and too enthusiastic a resection of the levator will cause what amounts to a cicatricial entropion whether the resection is anterior or posterior and no matter how small the conjunctival loss. Needless to say, wholesale resection or destruction of tarsoconjunctiva will cause entropion, as it did in the heyday of tarsal resection for trachoma. But, by and large, entropion in ptosis surgery is caused by resecting too much levator rather than conjunctiva.

The most common complication of levator surgery—anterior or posterior—is lid lag. Another common complaint is failure of the operated eye to close in sleep. What is sometimes forgotten is that lid lag is frequently a preexisting condition of congenital ptosis due to the levator dystrophy which caused the ptosis originally (Fig. 34A, B). It has also been shown statistically that about 2 per cent of Caucasian and 5 per cent of Chinese adults have physiologic lagophthalmos or eyes normally open in sleep. This is true of an even larger percentage of patients with ptosis. Hence the surgeon would be wise to inquire carefully into this *before* operation. He will be surprised to find how often a postoperative "complication" existed preoperatively. It is also well to remember that lid lag, unlike lagophthalmos, is not due to overcorrection but is inherent in the affection no matter how excellent the result.

In the case of young infants, in whom examination is difficult, to put it mildly, one can understand a surgeon's desire to postpone surgery to the time when more factual evidence is ascertainable about the type of ptosis and the amount of levator action. Some surgeons do levator resection in all cases and are successful in some because a hitherto unascertainable levator action was present. Other surgeons prefer to do a frontalis suspension procedure when the true nature of the ptosis cannot be determined; later, if levator action proves to be present, the frontalis sling is rather easily undone and a levator resection substituted. The reverse is, of course, even simpler. If levator resection proves unsuccessful, frontalis suspension can always be done. The decision will depend on the surgeon's power of observation and, in the last analysis, on his experience.

Tarsectomy

FASANELLA-SERVAT PROCEDURE (MODIFIED)

The Fasanella-Servat technic with the modification I suggested several years ago is useful where levator action is good and minimal levator shortening is needed. In general, its value is limited to traumatic and neurogenic ptosis such as Horner's syndrome. This is one of the few posterior approaches I occasionally use.

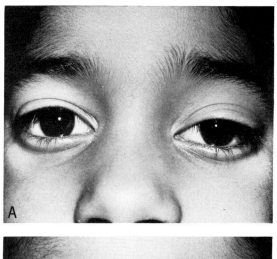

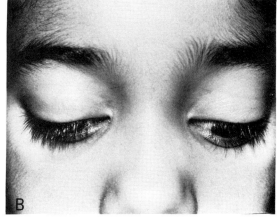

Fig. 34. Preoperative Lid Lag in Ptosis. *A.* Mild congenital ptosis of the left upper lid. *B.* Lid lag on looking down.

Surgical Technic (Fig. 35): The upper lid is everted and the doubled-up tarsus and conjunctiva are grasped in two small clamps. The clamps should be sufficiently posterior to the attached tarsal border to permit resection of 3 mm of doubled-up tissue and to allow easy suturing of the cut edges. The folded tarsus-cum-conjunctiva is resected (Fig. 35A). The wound is closed with a 5-0 plain catgut running suture with the knots placed well beyond the cornea on each side (Fig. 35B). The clamps are removed, the lid reinverted, ointment instilled, and a monocular patch applied. The dressing is changed daily and the cornea carefully inspected. Dressings are removed on the fifth or sixth day.

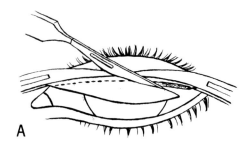

A

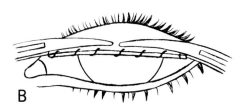

B

Fig. 35. Fasanella-Servat Technic of Ptosis Repair (Modified). *A.* The lid is everted and clamped as far posteriorly as possible. *B.* The wound is closed with a running suture knotted at each end beyond the cornea.

Comment: Lid elevation is due primarily to tarsal shortening here. Plain catgut and a running unknotted suture (except at each end) are used to minimize possible corneal irritation, since the suture is inevitably juxtaposed to the cornea. Plain catgut softens and absorbs readily and the running suture should contain only enough loops to ensure adequate closure. Despite all this the patient is usually assured of some discomfort the first few days.

Frontalis Suspension

When there is less than 2 mm of levator action, frontalis suspension is indicated. I have tried and given up all types of frontalis slings except autogenous fascia and, to a lesser extent, autogenous skin owing to the recurrences and complications encountered with heterografts.

FRONTALIS SUSPENSION BY AUTOGENOUS FASCIA SLING—AUTHOR'S METHOD

Obtaining Fascia (Fig. 36): The fascia strip is first obtained. After presurgical preparation of the area a 1.0- to 1.5-in horizontal skin incision is made in the lower outer aspect of the thigh. The incision is deepened through the subcutaneous fat down to the fascia lata. Bleeding is slight and easily controlled by pressure and a few ties. By means of long tonsil scissors the wound is undermined upward between the fat and fascia for about 4.0 to 4.5 inches (about 10 to 12 cm). A horizontal incision is made in the fascia, the fascia is raised, and the scissors are inserted *beneath* the fascia, which

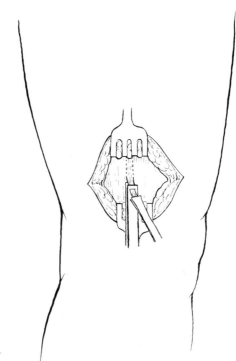

Fig. 36. Obtaining Autogenous Fascia. See text for details.

is again undermined upward for the same distance as anteriorly, in order to allow free and easy passage of the stripper.

A tongue of fascia 1 cm wide is made, threaded into a stripper, and held taut in a clamp; the stripper is moved upward cutting a strip of fascia about 12 cm long (Fig. 36). The thigh wound is closed with plain catgut subcuticular and a few interrupted silk skin sutures. A single-armed 5-0 silk suture is passed through each end of the fascia strip, knotted, and the needle cut off. A strip of fascia 8 to 10 mm wide and 12 cm long can be split vertically and suffices for bilateral repair.

Surgical Technic (Fig. 37): The brow and lid are now prepared for the reception of the autogenous fascia sling. Two 4-mm horizontal lid incisions are made 4 mm above the ciliary margin. One is placed at the junction of the medial and middle thirds and the other at the junction of the middle and lateral thirds of the lid. The incisions are carried through skin and muscle down to tarsus. Three similiar horizontal incisions are made just above the brow (Fig. 37A). One is placed centrally and the others about 15 mm to each side. These incisions are through the skin and muscle only. The middle brow incision is undermined upward under the skin and muscle for about 1 cm to create a pocket (Fig. 37C, *inset*).

A Reese ptosis knife or Wright needle is passed horizontally from one lid incision to the other between the tarsus and the orbicularis. As the

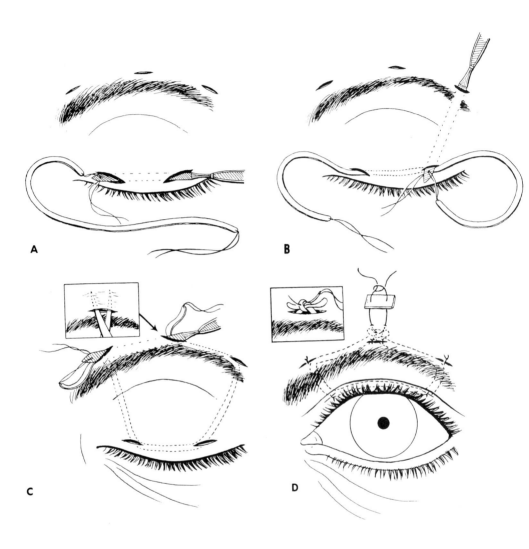

Fig. 37. Frontalis Suspension by Autogenous Fascia Sling—Author's Technic.
A. Two short incisions are made 4 mm above the lid margin and three incisions
above the brow. The fascia strip is pulled through the two lid incisions. B. The
strip is pulled up to the brow laterally and medially. C. The central brow incision is undermined upward (*inset*). Both ends of the fascia strip are pulled out
through the central brow incision. D. The ends of the fascia are tied and the
lid pulled up. The knot is reinforced with a chromic suture to prevent slippage
(*inset*). A 4-0 silk suture is passed through the knot without tying and into the
pocket above the central incision to emerge on the skin surface about 1 cm above
the brow. The suture is tied over a peg and the incisions are closed. (From Fox,
S. A. *J. Pediatr. Ophthalmol.* 61:522, 1966.)

fenestrated end of the knife emerges, the suture is threaded through it (Fig. 37A) and the fascia strip is drawn back so that it lies between the two lid incisions. The strip is not sutured to the tarsus. The Reese knife is now passed under the skin and muscle from the lateral brow incision to emerge in the lateral lid incision. The lateral suture is threaded into it and the fascia strip (Fig. 37B) is drawn upward to emerge above the brow. The medial end of the fascia strip is drawn up in similar fashion to emerge through the medial brow incision.

The knife is now passed from the middle to the lateral brow incision and the fascia strip is drawn through to emerge in the middle incision above the brow (Fig. 37C). The medial end of the fascia strip is drawn through the middle brow incision similarly. The two ends of the fascia are knotted and tightened so that the margin of the lid is drawn up some-what above the upper limbus to allow for the usual subsequent sagging. Care must be taken not to overcorrect lest notching result. The fascia is double-knotted and a 4-0 chromic suture is passed through the knot and tied to prevent loosening of the slippery fascia (Fig. 37D, inset). The excess fascia is resected, a double-armed 4-0 silk suture is passed through the knot without tying, and the needles are passed upward into the previously made pocket to emerge on the skin surface about 1 cm above the middle brow incision. The suture is tied over a rubber peg (Fig. 37D).

In the case of a young child, the brow incisions are closed with 4-0 or 5-0 plain catgut. The lid incisions need not be sutured. However, if sutures are desired, they should be inserted before the lid is pulled up and while the incisions are still easily accessible.

A modified Frost suture is passed through the lower lid, which is pulled up over the cornea, and the suture is taped to the brow with adhesive. Rarely does the Frost suture have to be left in more than 2 or 3 days because the operated lid becomes heavy and edematous and hangs over the cornea for several days. On the sixth day the skin sutures and patch are removed. The central brow suture is left in for 4 or 5 more days to assure proper support to the lid during healing.

FRONTALIS SUSPENSION WITH AUTOGENOUS SKIN SLING—AUTHOR'S METHOD

This procedure is useful when the lids are of normal width (they are not always so in congenital ptosis) and when, for some reason, obtaining fascia from the thigh is inconvenient or interdicted. Unlike a muscle sling, skin does not stretch much and hence works as well and as long as a fascia sling. Furthermore, the patient is spared a secondary operation and a scar on the thigh.

Surgical Technic (Fig. 38): With an antiseptic dye a horizontal line is marked out on the skin surface from canthus to canthus about 5 mm above the lid border. A second line, parallel with the first, is drawn 5 mm above.

If infiltration anesthesia has been used, the lid is gently massaged to reduce anesthetic swelling. An Ehrhardt clamp is inserted under the

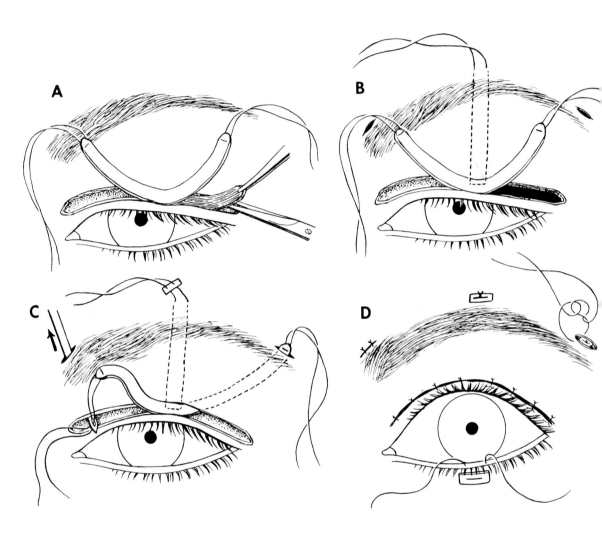

Fig. 38. Frontalis Suspension with Autogenous Skin—Author's Technic. *A.* A 5-mm wide strip of skin is raised 5 mm above the lid margin. It is left attached in the center. Sutures are inserted at each end of the strip. The exposed orbicularis muscle fibers are resected. *B.* Incisions are made above the medial and lateral ends of the brow about 15 mm from the center. A 3-0 silk suture is passed through tarsus under the central attachment of the skin strip, then upward, behind the orbicularis, to emerge above the brow. *C.* The de-epithelialized skin strips are drawn up medially and laterally beneath the orbicularis. *D.* The central suture is tied and the lid drawn up. The skin flaps are tautened into position. A Frost suture is placed in the lower lid to be drawn up for corneal coverage. (From Fox, S. A. *Am. J. Ophthalmol.* 65:359, 1968.)

lid and the skin incised along the marked-out lines except for the central 6 mm, which is left intact. The exposed orbicularis fibers are resected (Fig. 38A). The straps must be long enough to reach under the brow.

The skin flaps are smoothed out, epithelial side up, over a sheet of plastic or gauze and painted with 33% trichloracetic acid which is left on for 2 or 3 minutes. Care is taken that the surrounding tissue is well protected (although I have never seen anything drastic happen when a few drops of diluted acid are spilled accidentally). As the acid is applied, the skin surface turns grayish white. The epithelium is scraped off with a knife, and the straps are wiped and flushed off with saline. The skin retains its gray color but this is of no consequence. A single-armed 5-0 silk suture is passed through the end of each strap and the needles are cut off (Fig. 38A).

Small incisions are made through skin and muscle above the brow about 15 mm medial and lateral to the center. The central part of the lid between the brow and the lid incision is undermined beneath the orbicularis. A stout double-armed 3-0 silk suture is passed through the center of the lid engaging the orbicularis and tarsus beneath the area of attachment of the skin pedicles. The needles are carried up behind the orbicularis and are passed deep into the muscle layer of the brow to come out above the brow (Fig. 38B).

A Reese ptosis knife or Wright needle is passed deep under the brow through the temporal incision and behind the orbicularis to emerge at the point of attachment of the lateral skin pedicle. The instrument is moved from side to side to assure a sufficiently wide tunnel to permit passage of the pedicle. The suture attached to the lateral skin pedicle is threaded through the fenestrated end and the pedicle drawn up into the lateral brow wound. The medial pedicle is drawn up similarly (Fig. 38C).

The lid is drawn up by means of the central suture to a point slightly above the limbus, and the suture is tied securely over a peg. The medial and lateral pedicles are then drawn up, the lid margin is inspected to assure proper curve and position, and the pedicle ends are sutured subcutaneously. The lid and brow wounds are closed with interrupted sutures of 5-0 silk or, in a young patient, 5-0 plain catgut (Fig. 38D).

In closing the lid wound, four equally spaced sutures are placed along the length of the wound as follows: Each suture is passed through the lower lip of the wound, the upper tarsal border, then the upper wound lip. These sutures help restore the normal lid fold anatomy. Additional skin-to-skin sutures are added for good closure. A modified Frost suture is inserted in the lower lid which is drawn up over the cornea and taped to the forehead.

The eye is dressed daily and the silk sutures are removed on the sixth day. The central brow suture is left in for at least 10 to 12 days.

Comment: Since the skin straps are completely covered there is no burrowing of skin pedicles under surface skin and no redundant skin pockets; hence a presentable lid fold results. It must be emphasized that this operation cannot be used in congenitally narrowed lids which do not have ample skin.

Hildreth and Silver have suggested a Supramid sling for frontalis suspension which is inserted *under* the periosteum of the orbital rim. They feel that this is a better physiologic approach to frontalis suspension. However, since their sutures are passed *under* the periosteum, which is an immovable tissue closely applied to the bone, logically, movement of the frontalis would be aided very little and would probably be impeded.

The controversy about whether to do bilateral frontalis suspension in a patient with monocular ptosis for the purpose of cosmetic symmetry still simmers. Such a procedure, of course, gives bilateral lid lag on looking down and bilateral ptosis on looking up. Since lid lag is not uncommon after levator resection, such pursuit of symmetry would logically demand that all patients with monocular ptosis should have bilateral operations. The imagination boggles.

CONTRAINDICATIONS TO FRONTALIS SUSPENSION

There are several situations in which frontalis suspension should be used with great circumspection:

1. In strabismus fixus
2. In the absence of Bell's reaction
3. In cases of weak orbicularis action with poor lid closure

Since the eye is usually partially open after any frontalis suspension operation, an eye which fails to roll up enough leaves the cornea exposed and may suffer irreparable damage. In all such cases the better part of valor is discretion.

REFERENCES

Beard, C. Ptosis: Some newer concepts. *Ann. Ophthalmol.* 3:1047, 1971.

Duke-Elder, S. *Text-Book of Ophthalmology.* St. Louis, Mosby, 1952.

Fasanella, R. M., and Servat, J. Levator resection for minimal ptosis: Another simplified operation. *Arch. Ophthalmol.* 65:493, 1961.

Fox, S. A. Congenital ptosis: Frontalis sling. *J. Pediatr. Ophthalmol.* 61:522, 1966.

Fox, S. A. A new frontalis skin sling. *Am. J. Ophthalmol.* 65:359, 1968.

Fox, S. A. *Surgery of Ptosis.* Grune & Stratton, New York, 1968, p. 80.

Fox, S. A. Progressive familial myopathic ptosis. *Ann. Ophthalmol.* 3:1033, 1971.

Fuchs, A., and Wu, F. C. Sleep with half open eyes (physiologic lagophthalmos). *Am. J. Ophthalmol.* 31:717, 1948.

Gunn, R. M. Congenital ptosis with peculiar associated movements of the affected lids. *Trans. Ophthalmol. Soc. U.K.* 3:283, 1883.

Hildreth, H. R., and Silver, B. Physiologic approach to frontalis lid suspension. *Trans. Am. Acad. Ophthalmol. Otolaryngol.* 74:427, 1970.

Howitt, D. A., and Goldstein, J. H. Physiologic lagophthalmos. *Am. J. Ophthalmol.* 68:355, 1969.

Iliff, C. E. *Surgical Management of Ptosis.* Ethicon, Somerville, 1963.

Iliff, C. E. The optimum time for surgery in the Marcus Gunn phenomenon. *Trans. Am. Acad. Ophthalmol. Otolaryngol.* 74:1005, 1970.

Kestenbaum, A. *Clinical Methods of Neuro-Ophthalmogic Examination.* New York, Grune & Stratton, 1946, p. 308.

Kuhn, R., and Romano, P. E. Blepharoptosis, blepharophimosis, epicanthus inversus, and telecanthus: Syndrome with no name. *Am. J. Ophthalmol.* 72: 625, 1971.

Laughlin, R. G. Congenital fibrosis of the extraocular muscles. *Am. J. Ophthalmol.* 41:432, 1956.

Victor, M., Hayes, R., and Adams, R. D. Oculopharyngeal muscular dystrophy. *N. Engl. J. Med.* 267:1267, 1962.

Waardenburg, P. J., Franceschetti, A., and Klein, D. Oxford, *Genetics in Ophthalmology* Vol. 1, Blackwell, Scientific Publications, 1961, p. 415.

CHAPTER 5

Ectropion

SURGERY OF SENILE ECTROPION

I wish I could say that the last few years have produced startlingly new and significant information about the etiology and treatment of senile ectropion; but they have not. Current concepts of treatment have pretty well ruled out lid splitting, and senile ectropion is now repaired by means of the old technics of Blaskovics and Imré with, of course, the inevitable modifications, some of which are important.

Our understanding of the causes of senile ectropion is *in statu quo*. We have long known that senile ectropion (and entropion) of the lower lid are products of the aging process during which mesodermal tissues shrink. The panniculus adiposus is slowly absorbed, muscle tissue becomes flabby and stringy, and the bones lose their calcium and grow brittle. As a result, the body's ectodermal envelope becomes too large for its contents and begins to show bags and folds and wrinkles. Hence senile ectropion is due to the slow but inevitable progressive atonia and relaxation of all the lid tissues: skin, muscle, fascia, conjunctiva, and tarsal sling (the tarsus with its two tough canthal ligaments). Its development is marked by a syndrome of events which come on gradually and tend to merge into each other:

1. Loss of tonus with tissue relaxation
2. Eversion
3. Elongation
4. Sagging
5. Conjunctival hypertrophy and keratinization

Surgery for senile ectropion must be adapted to the particular stage of its development. At the onset of the ectropic evolution relatively mild measures will suffice. As the ectropion becomes more severe, the surgery required becomes more elaborate.

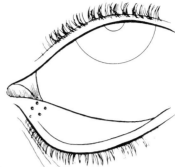

Fig. 39.   Cautery Puncture for Punctal Eversion.

Loss of Tonus and Relaxation

In early ectropion, even before eversion becomes obvious, the relaxation and atonia of the lid are sometimes enough to embarrass tear conduction. For although the lid may appear to be in normal position, the close apposition of the punctum to the globe has been relaxed and tearing may result. Here some benefit may be gained by a localized cautery puncture below the punctal area.

LOCALIZED CAUTERY PUNCTURE

Surgical Technic (Fig. 39): The medial portion of the lid is everted and a few drops of lidocaine are injected subconjunctivally beneath the punctum. With a fine hot muscle hook two rows of two punctures each are laid down below the punctum sufficiently low so that there is no danger of injury to the canaliculus. After healing and cicatrization this may cause enough inversion of the punctum to stop tearing.

MEDIAL CONJUNCTIVOPLASTY

A small horizontal conjunctivoplasty below the punctal area works just as well as the cautery puncture and may be preferable in some cases.

Surgical Technic (Fig. 40): After local infiltration of anesthetic a horizontal spindle of conjunctiva and subjacent fascia measuring 4 by 8 mm is resected 5 mm below the punctum and sutured (Fig. 40). This procedure, like the cautery puncture, causes punctal inversion and may suffice until the ectropic process starts to evert the lid again—as it will.

Eversion

MEDIAL TARSORRHAPHY—ARLT'S METHOD

As medial eversion increases and the punctum emerges from its hidden position against the globe, more definitive treatment becomes neces-

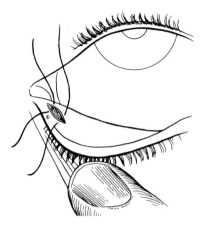

Fig. 40. Conjunctivoplasty for Punctal Eversion.

sary. The medial tarsorrhaphy was used by Arlt 150 years ago to repair eversion of the medial portion of the lower lid and the punctum in early ectropion. It was also used when an old enucleation had produced shelving of the lower lid with inability to retain a prosthesis.

Surgical Technic (Fig. 41): The procedure consists of the resection of a narrow strip of epithelium all around the margin of the medial canthus nasal to the upper and lower puncta. To ensure a permanent result two rows of sutures should be laid down. The inner lips of the upper and lower wounds are closed with a running suture of 6-0 chromic catgut. The outer lips are closed with interrupted sutures of 5-0 or 6-0 silk. The latter are removed on the fifth or sixth day after operation.

MEDIAL CANTHOPLASTY

When the lower lid is extremely lax it may be necessary to do a small canthoplasty. This is also used to help bolster a more elaborate ectropion repair (see below).

Surgical Technic (Fig. 42): The lid margins medial to the puncta are freshened as for tarsorrhaphy and the posterior lips of the wound are sewn together with 6-0 chromic catgut. A rectangle of skin about 8 to 10 mm in width is then resected from the upper lid and a skin sliding flap of equal size is fashioned in the lower lid. The flap is pulled up to cover the bared area in the upper lid and sutured into position with interrupted 6-0 silk sutures.

Comment: Since, like the lateral tarsorrhaphy, this procedure narrows as well as shortens the palpebral fissure, it can also be used to relieve advanced exophthalmos as an adjunct to lateral canthoplasty.

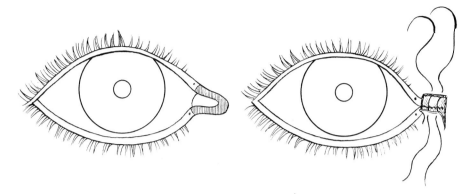

Fig. 41. Simple Medial Tarsorrhaphy—Arlt's Method.

Fig. 42. Simple Medial Canthoplasty.

Medial canthal surgery is sometimes employed in unusual types of ectropion as a method of desperation. Pictured in Figure 43A is a patient with leontiasis ossea whose lower lids are so lax that even in closure they hang down exposing the caruncle and plica (Fig. 43B). An ectropion repair did not suffice and medial canthal surgery was needed (Fig. 43C) to attain closure of the palpebral fissures (Fig. 43D). This is one of the rare instances in which this type of tarsorrhaphy is justified.

To sum up then, indications for a medial tarsorrhaphy or canthoplasty include (1) advanced exophthalmos in which lateral tarsorrhaphy furnishes insufficient corneal protection, (2) unusually lax lower lids which are not responsive to ordinary ectropion reparative technics, and (3) lower medial punctum eversion not repairable by other methods of reinversion. Since the permanent medial tarsorrhaphy covers plica and caruncle (Fig. 43C) and hence constitutes a cosmetic blemish, it should be used sparingly and only when other methods are contraindicated or have failed.

Eversion and Elongation

As medial eversion progresses, elongation sets in and not only must the punctum be reinverted but the lid must be shortened. This fact did not escape the notice of the keen clinicians of an earlier day and they proceeded to the surgical correction of the ectropic lid with enthusiasm and fervor. It is in this connection that we first meet the immortal full-thickness base-up triangle—immortal because, despite numerous burials, it has refused to stay dead.

The earliest report of resection of a base-up, full-thickness triangle to correct lengthening of the ectropic lid was that of Adams in 1812. He resected the triangle "about a quarter inch from the external angle of the lower lid." von Ammon (1831) did the same *at* the lateral canthus (Fig. 44A). Lawrence (1854) moved the site of resection to "about an inch" from

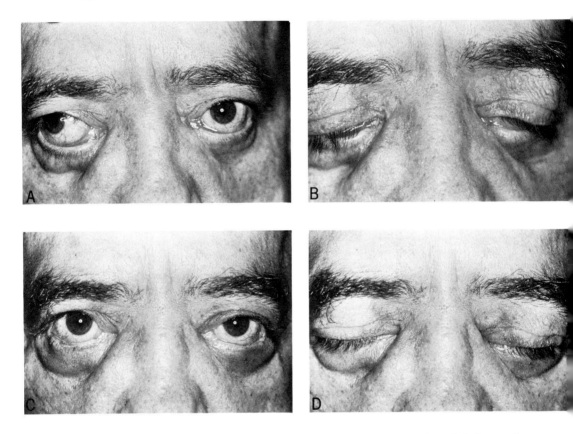

Fig. 43. Ectropion in Leontiasis Ossea. *A.* Ectropion and lagophthalmos of both lower lids. *B.* The lower lids are still lagophthalmic on closure. *C.* Appearance after correction. *D.* Closure is now complete.

the lateral canthus. Davis (1911) revived the procedure again as a "new principle" and sutured the cut tarsus to the periosteum (Fig. 44*B*). Molnar (1962) resected the triangle as Adams did. Bick (1966) exhumed the von Ammon procedure under the rather grandiloquent title of "orbital tarsal disparity" (Fig. 44*C*), and Leone in 1970 reported suturing the cut tarsus to the periosteum as Davis did.

    Thus the identical procedure has been revived and rediscovered over the years some half dozen times and has pursued the hapless lid relentlessly. But each time, the procedure died. It died because it does not do what its succession of rediscoverers say it does. From its inception the main trouble with the lateral full-thickness triangle resection technic was its failure to achieve complete inversion of the *whole* lid in ectropion of any degree. The cosmetic result is almost always good, but the procedure is seldom successful in attaining complete inversion at the punctum.

    Various attempts, short of direct surgery in the punctal area, were made. But it was not until Kuhnt in 1883 resurrected the old Antyllus lid-

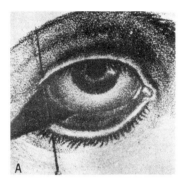
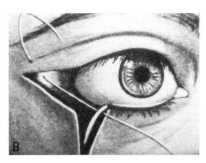
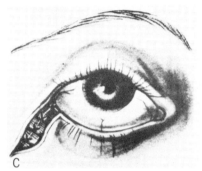

Fig. 44. Full-Thickness Base-Up Triangle Resections. A. von Ammon's Method. B. Davis' Method. C. Bick's Method.

splitting operation of the seventh century that a partial solution was obtained. Splitting the lid and resecting tarsoconjunctiva as close as possible to the punctum gives a much better result than a simple lateral or even central wedge resection. For the further the resection is from the medial canthus the poorer the punctal inversion, and the nearer the resection is medially, the better the reinversion. The trouble is that lid splitting is objectionable not only because it jeopardizes cilia but because it does not produce adequate punctal inversion in advanced senile ectropion. For, as everybody knows, the punctal area remains stubborn and, while a good cosmetic result is usually obtainable with lid shortening, inversion and cessation of tearing are much more difficult to attain. No wonder lid splitting is gradually disappearing here as everywhere.

Obviously the medial canthus must receive more and more attention as the severity of the ectropion increases. Hence in advanced senile ectropion adjunctive medial surgery such as cautery (Fig. 39), tarsorrhaphy (Fig. 41), or even a medial ectropion repair (Fig. 45) may be necessary. In paralytic ectropion medial repair is always called for, as shown below.

MEDIAL ECTROPION REPAIR—BLASKOVICS' PROCEDURE (MODIFIED)

In 1938 Blaskovics published a procedure for ectropion repair at the medial canthus. I have used this—in modified form—with satisfaction for moderate atonic ectropion with lid lengthening (Fig. 45D).

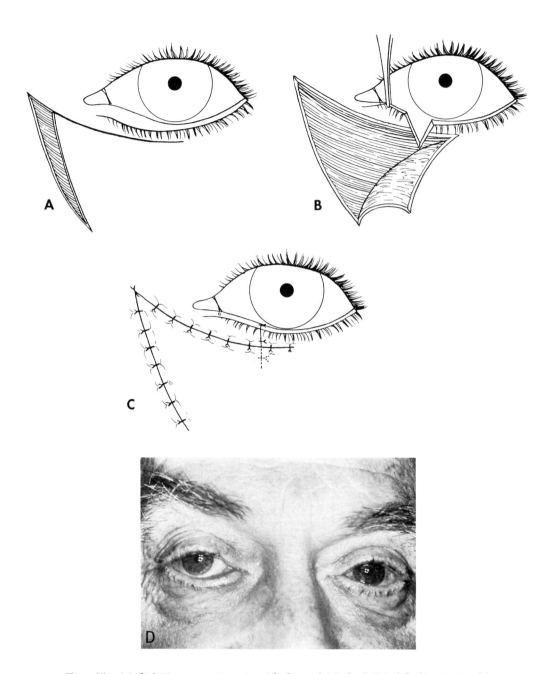

Fig. 45. Medial Ectropion Repair—Blaskovics' Method (Modified). *A.* A skin incision is made below the medial half of the lower lid and carried up and nasally. A narrow skin triangle is resected in the nasocanthal angle. *B.* The skin flap is undermined laterally, and a full-thickness triangle, base-up, is resected about 5 mm from the punctum. *C.* The triangular wound is closed in layers. An intermarginal (figure-8) suture is optional. The skin flap is drawn up, any further skin excess is resected, and the wound is closed. *D.* Bilateral senile ectropion. *E.* (*opposite page*) Appearance before suture removal. *F.* (*opposite page*) Final result. (From Fox, S. A. *Arch. Ophthalmol.* 80:494, 1968.)

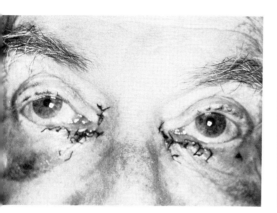
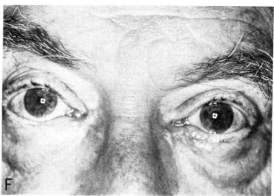

Surgical Technic (Fig. 45): A horizontal skin incision is made below the medial half of the lower lid 4 mm from the lid margin. The incision is carried upward and nasally following the curve of the lower lid. A narrow triangle of skin is resected in the nasocanthal angle (Fig. 45A). The skin is undermined laterally and the skin flap is mobilized. The lid is folded over to allow estimation of the amount of lengthening, and the excess of full-thickness lid is resected triangularly, apex downward, about 5 mm lateral to the punctum (Fig. 45B). The triangular lid wound is sutured anteriorly and posteriorly. The skin flap is drawn nasally, any further skin excess is resected, and the wound is closed (Fig. 45C). Figure 45E shows the appearance before suture removal and Figure 45F the final result.

Comment: This procedure usually produces good inversion of the punctum without covering the plica or the caruncle. There are two important modifications of the original Blaskovics procedure in this technic: (1) the skin incision is made close to the lid margin where the scar is inconspicuous, and (2) a triangle instead of a rectangle is resected from the lower lid, allowing easier and better cosmetic closure and better inversion of the ectropic lower lid.

Only enough skin must be resected to cause the lid to lie snugly against the globe and to invert the punctum. Too much resection may produce a cicatricial epicanthal fold which is not easy to correct.

This procedure is well adapted for all cases of moderate ectropion with eversion and not too much elongation. The punctal eversion is corrected by the shortening and pulling of the skin flap upward and medially. In advanced ectropion, this procedure is not quite adequate because of space limitations at the nasocanthal angle; hence one must resort to the lateral canthal angle.

Eversion, Elongation, and Sagging of the Lid

When eversion and lid lengthening have proceeded still further, considerable sagging of the lid is added. The problem at this stage is not only to invert and shorten the lid but also to hang it back up in its normal position. Dieffenbach (1848) tried to do this by resecting a skin triangle beyond the lateral canthus and pulling the lid straight out. However, it was not until Szymanowski (1870) reported his method of pulling the lid *up* as well as out that the problem was satisfactorily solved. This Szymanowski triangle in one form or another is probably the only important survivor of the many modifications of the once much-used Kuhnt-Szymanowski operation.

Today, the type of procedure which has replaced the classic Kuhnt-Szymanowski technic shuns lid splitting and requires resection of the full-thickness base-up triangle as close to the medial canthus as possible. Even here additional medial canthus surgery may be needed. The procedure that does this best is a modification of the Blaskovics operation.

LATERAL ECTROPION REPAIR—BLASKOVICS' PROCEDURE (MODIFIED)

Surgical Technic (Fig. 46): A horizontal skin incision is made along the outer half (more, if necessary) of the lower lid, 4 mm below the ciliary margin. The incision is carried up and out beyond the canthus following the lid curve. At the end of this incision a vertical 15-mm incision is made downward. The resultant skin flap is undermined and mobilized (Fig. 46A). A full-thickness triangle, apex-down, of excess lid tissue is resected as close to the medial end of the skin incision as possible (Fig. 46B). Enough full-thickness lid should be resected to make the closure snug and to correct the lengthening. The wound is closed in layers. An intermarginal figure-8 closure is optional. The skin flap is pulled up laterally and the excess resected (Fig. 46C). It is sutured into position with interrupted sutures of 5-0 silk (Fig. 46D). These skin sutures are removed on the fifth or sixth day, the notch sutures a couple of days later if they have not loosened earlier.

Comment: This procedure shortens the lid and pulls it up into its normal position. Occasionally the punctal area is not completely inverted. In such cases a few cautery punctures below the punctum (Fig. 39) or a conjunctivoplasty (Fig. 4D) will complete the repair. The recently suggested resection of a simple central full-thickness, apex-down wedge will not bring the lid margin up to its normal position any better in advanced senile ectropion; nor will the punctum be inverted. Only in very early cases of ectropion is this maneuver successful.

Hypertrophy and Keratinization of the Conjunctiva

When eversion has been of long duration, the conjunctiva becomes thickened and keratinized and takes on a beefy red color. This occurs in long-neglected senile or paralytic ectropion and in cicatricial ectropion of the old accompanied by much tearing with excoriation and contraction of the lower lid skin.

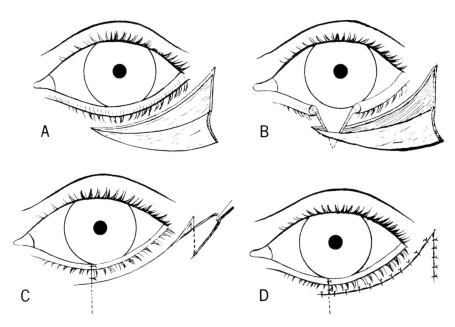

Fig. 46. Lateral Ectropion Repair—Blaskovics' Method (Modified). *A.* The skin is incised 4 mm below the lateral half of the lid margin and the incision carried upward beyond the canthus. A vertical 15-mm incision is made downward from the end of the first incision. The resultant triangular flap is undermined and dissected down. *B.* A full-thickness triangle, apex down, is resected close to the medial end of the incisions. *C.* The triangular wound is sutured in layers. (A figure-8 closure is optional). The skin flap is pulled up laterally and excess skin resected. *D.* The skin is closed with interrupted sutures of 5-0 silk. (From Fox, S. A. *Ann. Ophthalmol.* 4:225, 1972.)

TERSON'S CONJUNCTIVAL SPINDLE RESECTION

When the conjunctiva in an ectropic lid becomes so thick due to exposure that inversion of the lower lid is prevented no matter how much it is shortened, the thickened exposed conjunctiva must be resected. This is done in spindle-shaped fashion.

Surgical Technic (Fig. 47): After suitable anesthesia a strip of thickened conjunctiva extending the entire length of the lower lid is dissected out. The upper horizontal incision outlining the strip is somewhat below the level of the canaliculus and the lower incision is at the lower edge of the exposed conjunctival bulge. The resection is down to tarsus with the tarsus spared. The conjunctival wound is closed with interrupted sutures of catgut or silk (Fig. 47). One then proceeds immediately with the ectropion repair.

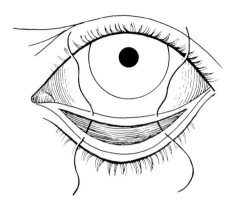

Fig. 47. Resection of Keratinized Conjunctiva—Terson's Method. A horizontal spindle of thickened conjunctiva is resected.

PARALYTIC ECTROPION

In paralytic ectropion the lid is completely atonic—to the extent that one wonders how a lid containing a tarsal plate can be so soft and flabby. Lagophthalmos is often associated because the lower lid does not always ride up enough for adequate closure. (Fig. 48B). A rather unusual characteristic of these paralytic lids is the absence of eversion; eversion may be present, however, and may vary from slight to extreme. If eversion is absent or mild (Fig. 48A), the usual modified Blaskovics procedure (Fig. 46) will suffice for repair. It may be quite enough (Fig. 48C) to bring the lid back into normal position (Fig. 48D) and effect adequate closure (Fig. 48E).

In complete atonic ectropion the lid often has to be shortened and pulled up both medially and laterally; the usual procedure (Fig. 46) alone will not suffice, and additional maneuvers must be employed. In all cases the modified Blaskovics procedure is done laterally. The punctal region will not be inverted. The medial procedure will then depend on the amount of reinversion necessary. If only slight reinversion is needed, cautery puncture will suffice. If more reinversion is required a medial tarsorrhaphy (Fig. 41) or a medial canthoplasty (Fig. 42) will have to be done. The medial sagging may be so marked as to demand ectropion correction medially (Fig. 45) as well as laterally.

CICATRICIAL ECTROPION—MILD

Cicatricial ectropion results from loss of superficial tissue, usually due to trauma but sometimes to cicatrizing skin conditions seen especially in older individuals. If the ectropion is of long duration, the conjunctiva may be thickened and require excision before inversion can be obtained. However,

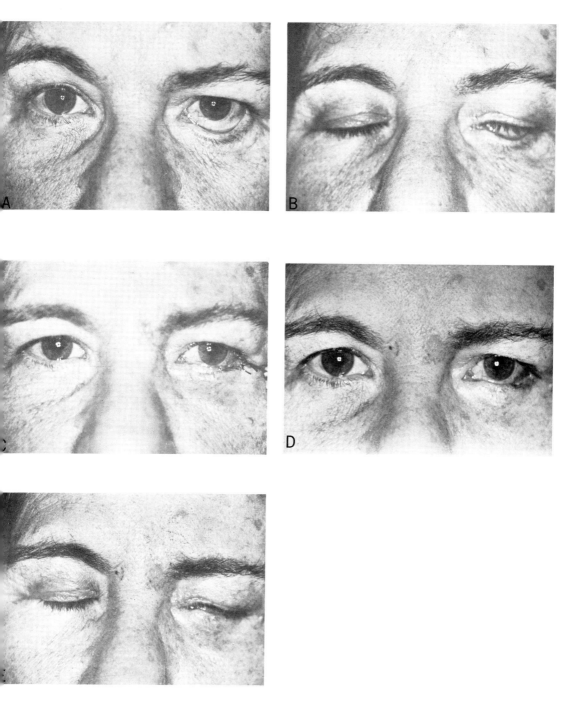

Fig. 48. Repair of Paralytic Ectropion of Left Lower Lid. *A* and *B*. Appearance with eye open and closed. *C.* Repair by lateral ectropion procedure. *D* and *E.* Postoperative appearance with eye open and shut.

simple inversion is rarely sufficient because the relative tissue proportion between skin and conjunctiva has been disturbed to such an extent by skin contraction that the skin loss must be restored in some way.

V-Y REPAIR—T. WHARTON JONES' METHOD

If the skin loss is minimal, enough relaxation may be obtained with a Z-plasty. If skin loss is somewhat greater, the V-Y-plasty of T. Wharton Jones may be employed to good purpose.

Surgical Technic (Fig. 49): A V incision is made below the lower lid. This must be generous enough to include the whole scarred area and some normal skin within its boundaries. The included skin is dissected up so that the lid border is in normal position against the globe. Any subcutaneous scar tissue encountered must be resected (Fig. 49A).

The wound edges are liberally undermined medially and laterally and closure is begun at the apex of the V with interrupted sutures. The suturing is carried upward as long as the wound edges can be brought together easily. Under no circumstances must the undermined skin flap be pulled down. It is sutured medially and laterally in its relaxed position. The wound closure has now assumed the figure of a Y with the length of the lower stalk depending on how much relaxation has been obtained (Fig 49B).

Comment: Overcorrection of cicatricial ectropion is welcome because the lid always tends to evert a little postoperatively. It cannot be overemphasized that the ectropion must be mild, for the V-Y technic will not work if an appreciable amount of skin has been lost. In the latter case,

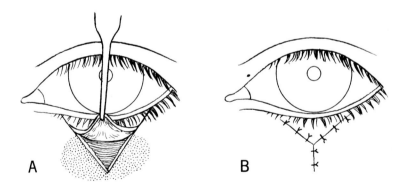

A   B

Fig. 49. V-Y Repair of Cicatricial Ectropion—Method of T. Wharton Jones. A. A V incision includes all the scarred lower lid tissue. The included skin is undermined to the lid margin. The adjacent skin is undermined medially and laterally (stippled area). B. Closure is begun at the apex and continued upward as long as the skin edges come together easily. It is then continued to form the arms of the Y.

skin grafting should be done at once with intermarginal sutures or surgical tarsorrhaphies (if the graft is large) to splint the lids and allow the wound to heal without contraction. (It is of interest to note that Wharton Jones recommended this technic for cicatricial ectropion of the *upper* lid where its success is considerably less than noteworthy. It is not advised.) The skin grafting procedure has been widely reported in numerous textbooks on ophthalmic surgery—including my own *Ophthalmic Plastic Surgery*, ed. 4.

REFERENCES

Adams, W. *Practical Observations on Ectropion.* London, Callow, 1812, pp. 4-6.

von Ammon, F. A. *Zeitschrift für die Ophthalmologie Verbindung mit vielen Aertzten.* Dresden, Walterschen Hof, 1830-1831, vol. IV, pp. 515-532.

Arlt, E. F. *Graefe-Saemisch Handbuch des gesamte Augenheilkunde.* Berlin, Reimer, 1841.

Bick, W. Orbital tarsal disparity. *Arch. Ophthalmol.* 75:386, 1966.

Blaskovics, L., and Kreiker, A. *Eingriffe aum Auge.* Stuttgart, Enke, 1938.

Davis, A. E. A new method in operating for ectropion. *J.A.M.A.* 57:1682, 1911.

Dieffenbach, J. F. *Die Operative Chirurgie.* Leipzig, Brockhaus, 1845-1848.

Fox, S. A. A medial ectropion procedure. *Arch. Ophthalmol.* 80:494, 1968.

Imré, J. Operation gegen Ektropium senile. *Klin. Monatsbl. Augenheilkde.* 95: 303, 1935.

Jones, T. W. *A Manual of the Principles and Practice of Ophthalmic Medicine and Surgery.* London, Churchill, 1847, pp. 413-429.

Kuhnt, H. *Beitrage zur Operationen Augenheilkunder.* Jena, Fischer, 1883, p. 45.

Lawrence, W. In I. Hays (ed.). *A Treatise of the Diseases of the Eye.* Philadelphia, Blanchard & Lea, 1854, vol. 18, p. 150.

Leone, C. R. Repair of ectropion using the Bick procedure. *Am. J. Ophthalmol.* 70:233, 1970.

Molnar, L. The revival of the 150-year-old operation of Adams. *Klin. Monatsbl. Augenheilkde.* 140:708, 1962.

Szymanowski, J. *Handbuch der Operationen Chirurgie.* Berlin, Braunschweig, 1870, p. 243.

Terson, A. Traitement l'ectropion sénile. *Arch. Ophtalmol.* 16:760, 1896.

Ziegler, S. L. Galvanocautery puncture in entropion and ectropion. *J.A.M.A.* 53:133, 1909.

CHAPTER 6

Entropion and Trichiasis

SENILE ENTROPION

Etiology

Senile entropion is as old as man, and its etiology has been an enigma for years. It has masqueraded under many names: organic, spasmodic, spastic, etc., etc. However, after many years of guesses and theories, some hard facts about its etiology have now emerged. These facts confirm some theories and dispose of others.

Of the many etiologic explanations, two have been especially hardy and long-lived even though not very convincing. The oldest is the "spastic" theory. Since the identity of its author or authors has been lost in the mist of years, this theory is apocryphal as well as unconvincing. For years it was accepted without question that some unexplained nerve reflex, mediated along some unknown sensory or motor nervous pathway, causes a spasm of the orbicularis with consequent entropion in older individuals. How this reflex is initiated and why it remains localized to the upper part of the lower lid has never been explained. Recently competent proof has been adduced that the entropion persists even when all sensory and motor nerve impulses to the lower lid are blocked. It has been shown that when the sensory nerves are anesthetized by instillation or infiltration to counteract all possible conjunctival irritation, the entropion persists (Fig. 50A); nor does akinesia cause the entropion to vanish (Fig. 50B). One wonders why the spastic theory has persisted so long, since it is so easily disproved. Although not as ancient, it is now one with Nineveh and Tyre. It should be.

Senile entropion should not be confused with spastic entropion. The latter is a transient condition caused by conjunctival irritation, acute ocular inflammation, or prolonged patching. Acute entropion may occur at any age, does not require surgery, and disappears when its cause is removed.

The second theory was proposed by Jones, Reeh, and Tsujimura in 1963. It casts the preseptal muscle as the villain in senile entropion by attributing to this luckless part of the orbicularis some strange and curious actions. This theory is not apocryphal, only unconvincing. This hypothesis admits a role for degenerative changes, but blames the entropion primarily on the preseptal muscle which, freeing itself from anterior skin and posterior

96

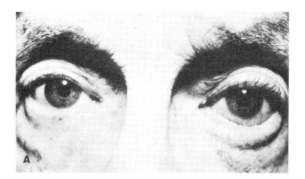

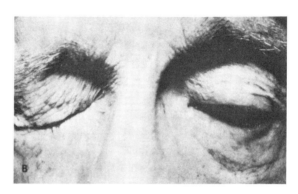

Fig. 50. Affect of Sensory and Motor Anesthesia on Senile Entropion. A. Senile entropion of the left lower lid. Instillation of anesthesia does not relieve the entropion. B. Akinesia leaves the entropic lid unaffected. (From Fox, S. A. *Ophthalmic Plastic Surgery*, ed. 4. New York, Grune & Stratton, 1970.)

fascial attachments in some unknown fashion, proceeds to creep up onto the tarsal surface, thus forcing the upper part of the lid to bend inward.

This concept ignores the anatomic fact that the preseptal muscle is an integral part of the orbicularis and occupies the central part of the muscle sheet. It is not a separate entity. We know that the orbicularis is a sphincter muscle which opens and shuts the lids to protect the globe. We also know that like all sphincters it consists of one sheet of circular muscle with a central opening, the palpebral fissure. The geographic division of this muscle sheet into pretarsal, preseptal, and preorbital portions is arbitrary and does not mean that the muscle consists of three separate entities. Hence for the preseptal muscle to creep up onto the tarsus, the central part of this flat muscle sheet would have to separate itself from overlying skin and underlying fascia and buckle up from its surroundings. How and why this would happen has never been explained; nor has such a muscle safari ever been seen by mortal eye.

Current experimental evidence has completely exploded the creeping preseptal theory. Dalgleish and Smith inserted metal markers into an entropic lid which had been pulled down and straightened as shown in Figure 51A. The two upper vertical markers are in the upper and lower tarsal borders, the two lower horizontal markers are in the preseptal fibers of the orbicularis. As the lid is allowed to resume its entropic position

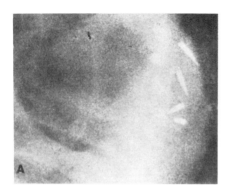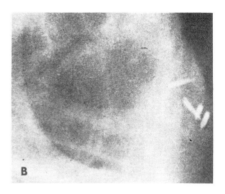

Fig. 51. X-Ray Study of Entropic Lid Action. A. Lower lid is pulled down into normal (nonentropic) position. The upper two vertical markers are in the upper and lower margins of the tarsal plate. The tarsus is between their two thickened ends. The two lower horizontal markers are in preseptal orbicularis. B. The same lid is now allowed to go back into its entropic position. The upper edge of the tarsus is now seen to be in a horizontal position and the lower margin has swung forward. It will be noted that the preseptal markers have approximated the lower tarsal border but they are nowhere near the anterior surface of the tarsus. (From Dalgleish, R., and Smith, J. L. S. *Br. Med. J.* 50:79-91, 1966.)

(Fig. 51B) the upper tarsal border is seen to turn in, the lower border swings out, and the pretarsal markers are pulled up by the curved-in tarsus. But note that the preseptal fibers are *not* pulled up on to the anterior surface of the tarsus. Despite such convincing proof ophthalmologists who should know better continue to pay obeisance to the myth of the creeping preseptal muscle.

What then is the mechanism of senile entropion? All the evidence we have now points to the simple and obvious anatomic fact of degenerative changes in senile entropion—as in ectropion—and away from unproved spasms and inexplicable gyrations of a fractious and fractionated orbicularis.

It is important to remember that senile entropion and ectropion are alike in many ways. The most important similarity is the atonicity and increased laxity of the lids in both affections. On the other hand, the most important difference is the condition of the tarsal sling, which has given way in senile ectropion but has retained its firmness and position in senile entropion. Thus in entropion the lid margin lies snugly—too snugly—against the globe, but the attached tarsal border has swung outward because of the laxity of tissues which normally hold the whole lid against the globe. With the upper tarsal border tight against the globe and the attached border loose, the lid curves in as it rises on blinking, and entropion is the result. The process is aided by the fact that the lower lid tarsus is narrower, thinner, and weaker than the upper lid tarsus. Upper lid senile entropion does not occur because the tarsus is too wide and thick.

Surgery to Correct Entropion

Surgical correction of atonic entropion of the lower lid has been of two schools: (1) by unwinding and (2) by wall strengthening. The former method is by far the older.

Unwinding the entropic lid or shortening it vertically by cautery or resection of horizontal strips of one, some, or all the lower lid tissues probably dates back to the Medes and Persians; it is certainly one of the earliest recorded lid procedures. It has the disadvantage of pulling the lid down and exposing sclera below the limbus.

Cauterization to unroll and evert the lid was probably first practiced by the ancient Egyptians and later by the Arabs. More recently thermo- or galvanocautery has been substituted. Celsus gets the credit for the simplest and earliest type of correction of entropion by resection of horizontal strips of tissue. Paulus of Aegina is said to have devised a special forceps for the operation. Inclusion of orbicularis muscle along with the skin excision was frequently practiced. Later canthotomy and cantholysis were added. Caustics such as sulfuric acid and potash were also used. Sutures have an old, honorable, and most ineffective history to which the names of many illustrious ophthalmologists are attached. Collodion and adhesive strips have no permanent value. All these maneuvers shorten the lid vertically and pull it down below the lower limbus to greater or lesser degree; the repair is impermanent.

Horizontal shortening of the lid by resection of *vertical* sections of lower lid tissue is a much later development. This tautens the lower lid and strengthens it without pulling it down. In the middle of the nineteenth century no great distinction was made between surgery for atonic (spasmodic, as it was then called) and for cicatricial entropion; or for that matter, between upper and lower lid surgery. (Resection of tissue triangles was first used by von Graefe for cicatricial entropion of the upper lid.) To compound confusion trichiasis was included in the procedures for all types of entropion since, it was said, "it is clinically impossible to separate trichiasis and entropion." Fortunately we know better now.

C. H. Beard later transferred von Graefe's triangular resection to the lower lid. Over 100 years ago resection of a triangle of skin at the lateral canthus was done with and without canthotomy. Horizontal fracture of the whole lid was done by Panas in 1882. This operation had numerous modifications.

Canthotomy and cantholysis do not relieve atonic entropion of long duration because the curved-in state of the tarsus has become chronic and remains constant unless the tarsal base is shortened and the tarsus thus tautened and everted. Shortening the *free* margin of the tarsus is unnecessary since this margin is already tightly up against the globe. It is the *attached tarsal* border, which has swung out, that needs tautening and shortening to reappose it to the globe. Hence any surgical procedure for atonic entropion must correct two conditions to be successful: (1) it must counteract by horizontal shortening the atonicity and stretching of the lid tissues which allow the lower tarsal border to swing out, and (2) it must prevent the outward roll of the attached border by shortening it.

In very early entropion external cautery puncture may help, but I have found it a temporary expedient frequently followed by recurrences, as Wheeler showed many years ago. A recent modification of my operation for senile entropion has proved entirely satisfactory and is described below. It has given me the least number of recurrences of any procedure I have used.

REPAIR OF SENILE ENTROPION—AUTHOR'S METHOD

Surgical Technic (Fig. 52): With an antiseptic dye a vertical spindle is outlined on the skin surface just beyond the lateral canthus. *The upper apex of the spindle is placed about 2 mm lateral to the lateral commissure and no higher.* The spindle is 10 to 15 mm wide at its widest point depending on the atonicity of the lid and how much tissue has to be resected. The lid is anesthetized and everted on a chalazion clamp. A triangle with its apex at the gray line and its base on the attached tarsal border is outlined with a knife just lateral to the center of the lid. The base measures 6 to 8 mm, again depending on the severity of the entropion and the amount to be resected (Fig. 52A). The tarsoconjunctival triangle is resected. It is not too important whether the apex of this triangle is at the lid margin or just below it, although I prefer the former location. The skin and muscle included within the spindle outline beyond the lateral canthus are resected (Fig. 52B). In severe entropion a spindle of orbital fascia is also resected.

The tarsal wound is closed with three or four interrupted sutures of 4-0 silk. The apex on the lid border may be closed with a 4-0 plain catgut suture. This suture sometimes irritates the lower cornea if the ends are left too long, but plain catgut softens rapidly and this suture has never been found to cause severe or prolonged irritation. If fascia has been resected laterally, this is closed first with 6-0 chromic catgut. The skin-muscle wound is closed with 5-0 silk sutures, care being taken to catch up the muscle fibers as well. Alternatively the muscle may be closed separately with 4-0 plain catgut (Fig. 52C) and then the skin with 5-0 silk (Fig. 52D).

Following surgery a firm supportive dressing is applied. The dressing is changed after 48 hours and then daily. Skin sutures are removed in 5 days and tarsal sutures in 10 days unless obviously loose before then.

Comment: The advantages of this technic are:
1. The surgery is quite simple.
2. It strengthens the tarsus, which is the only tough skeleton-like supportive structure of the lid. Since the tarsus does not stretch, recurrence of entropion is less frequent. Furthermore, the procedure shortens and strengthens the tarsus *at the base,* not at the apex, thus preventing the attached border from rolling out.
3. It also strengthens the other atonic tissues of the lid—the skin and muscle and, when necessary, the orbital fascia—not vertically

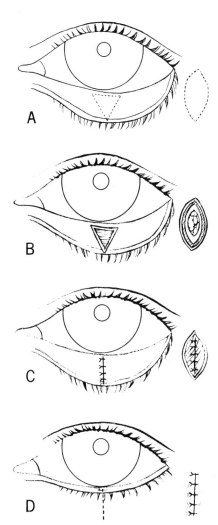

Fig. 52. Repair of Senile Entropion—Author's Technic. A. A vertical skin spindle is outlined just beyond the lateral canthus. The upper apex of the spindle is no higher than the lateral canthus. A tarsoconjunctival triangle with apex in the gray line and base on the attached tarsal border is outlined just lateral to the center of the lid. B. The included skin and muscle at the canthus are resected. Orbital fascia is also resected if entropion is severe. The outlined tarsoconjunctival triangle is resected. C. The tarsoconjunctival and lateral muscle wounds are closed. D. The skin at the lateral canthus is closed. See text for more details. (From Fox, S. A. Ann. Ophthalmol. 4:229, 1972.)

so as to pull the lid down, but horizontally to stiffen their support of the lid to the globe.

4. The only resultant scar is external to the lateral canthus where it is inconspicuous and gradually fades out.
5. If necessary the whole operation can be repeated.

In an earlier report it was suggested that a tarsoconjunctival triangle measuring no more than 5 or 6 mm at the base be resected. Later experience has proved this precaution unnecessary. Thus when the tarsus is unusually thin and the bulge severe, a 7- or 8-mm base-down triangle may be resected. Furthermore, immediate overcorrection is not catastrophic. In a couple of weeks all postoperative overcorrections tend to right themselves and disappear. In only two instances have a few Ziegler punctures been necessary to counteract an overcorrection.

On closure a small bump sometimes forms at the lid margin where the tarsal triangle has been resected. This disappears within 7 to 10 days.

Resection of the exposed orbital fascia laterally lends additional strength to the procedure. If orbital fat is exposed and prolapses, it is simply resected (to the cosmetic benefit of the patient, it might be added).

Undercorrection is possible and should be repaired on the operating table immediately if noted. An additional 2 or 3 mm of tarsus should be resected from one side of the tarsoconjunctival wound.

Since any operation for senile entropion can only treat the results of the aging process and not the cause, there will probably always be some recurrences. Hence the true value of any operation depends on the frequency of recurrences. In my experience the above procedure has given the least. The fact that the operation may be easily repeated enhances its value.

In recent years modifications have been reported in the literature proposing that rectangles of tarsus be resected instead of apex-up triangles. Since the upper border of the entropic lid is up tight against the globe and since it is the lower border of the tarsus which swings out, it seems to me more logical to tighten the *attached* border rather than the whole tarsus by triangular rather than rectangular resection.

Those who have used the above procedure over the years will note that the lateral triangle has again become a spindle; but *the upper apex of the spindle should lie opposite the lateral canthus and not higher*. This change has been made for two reasons:

1. The widest resection of skin and muscle is now in the center of the lower lid where it is most needed.
2. This gives a simpler closure with no skin wrinkling and less scarring; hence it is more acceptable cosmetically.

CICATRICIAL ENTROPION

Current concepts of cicatricial entropion have not changed materially. Cicatricial entropion, of course, is the reverse condition of cicatricial ectropion. The skin has remained intact but some of the tarsal and/or conjunctival lining of the lid has been lost, causing an inversion of the lid margin. It is usually due to conjunctival and tarsal cicatrization by trauma or disease, and correction requires restoration of the relative balance between skin and conjunctiva with the conjunctiva in this case requiring the restoration.

Lower Lid Entropion

The lower lid is somewhat simpler to repair than the upper lid because it is narrower and smaller. However, I have rarely seen a case of cicatricial entropion which can be permanently cured by external cautery

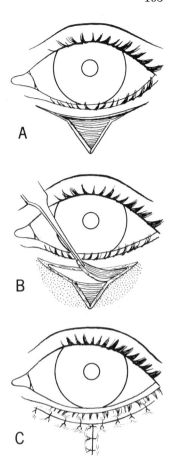

Fig. 53. Repair of Cicatricial Entropion of the Lower Lid—von Graefe's Method (Modified). *A.* A horizontal incision is made below the lid margin and a central skin triangle is resected below the incision. *B.* Orbicularis fibers are resected and the triangular wound lips undermined. *C.* Closure is made with interrupted silk sutures.

puncture. The everting potential of this relatively mild technic is just not enough.

REPAIR OF LOWER LID ENTROPION—VON GRAEFE'S METHOD (MODIFIED)

A modification of the old von Graefe (1864) technic is probably the most successful of the procedures for repair of lower lid cicatricial entropion. Enough skin should be resected to counterbalance tarsoconjunctival loss.

Surgical Technic (Fig. 53): A skin incision extending nearly the whole length of the lower lid is made 3 mm from and parallel with the free border. Two converging skin incisions are made downward, using the first incision as a base, and are placed so as to outline a central triangle with the apex down in the center of the lid. The size of this triangle will depend on how much correction is desired. Naturally the more tissue excised, the greater the everting effect will be. The triangle of skin is excised (Fig. 53A) and, if necessary, a 5-mm horizontal strip of orbicularis may also be resected the whole length of the wound to enhance the everting effect. The skin on each side is undermined (Fig. 53B) and the vertical wound is closed with

interrupted sutures of 5-0 silk. The horizontal wound is then closed similarly (Fig. 53C).

A firm dressing is applied for 2 days. The wound is dressed daily
thereafter and the sutures removed on the fifth or sixth day.

Comment: Since the horizontal skin incision is only 3 mm from the
ciliary margin, the result of this operation is to bring additional pressure
on the base of the tarsus and cause eversion of its margin. Although one
of the oldest, this is perhaps the best of the procedures using skin and
muscle excision for the correction of cicatricial entropion of the lower lid.
If the tissue loss is large, mucous membrane grafting will be necessary.
Tarsal fracture usually produces overcorrection and is better reserved for
the upper lid.

Upper Lid Entropion

Cicatricial entropion of the upper lid poses a considerably greater
surgical problem. The tarsus is longer and wider so that its roughening
and thickening gives more distortion. Also more conjunctiva has usually
been lost here. The decision whether to resect skin or graft conjunctiva
depends on *how much* tissue has been lost, where and at what expense to
the lid.

In olden days, when trachomatous entropion was common, resection
of the thick and distorted tarsoconjunctiva followed by grafting of healthy
mucous membrane was a common and successful procedure. Currently
trachoma is rare, but traumatic cicatricial entropion of the upper lid is
not unknown. The same procedure that is useful in lower lid inversion
due to lye burns (a not uncommon industrial and social trauma), is applicable to the upper lid. However, if the loss is not extreme, horizontal
section of the whole upper lid, an operation first suggested by Panas and
recently modified, has worked well.

HORIZONTAL TARSAL SECTION

Burow in 1873 was apparently the first to report complete horizontal
section of the tarsus. He included orbicularis and sometimes even skin.
Modifications soon followed. Panas' procedure of full-thickness lid section
has recently been modified and improved; it has become known as the
Wies procedure in the lower lid and the Ballen procedure in the upper lid.
Figure 54A illustrates cicatricial entropion of the upper lid repaired by this
technic.

Surgical Technic (Fig. 54): After suitable anesthesia an incision
through the full-thickness of the upper lid is made 4 mm above the lash

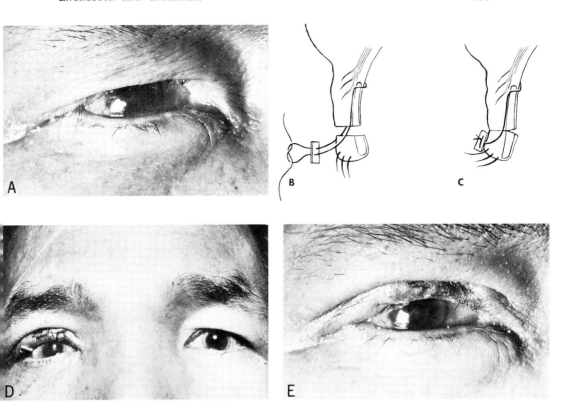

Fig. 54. Repair of Cicatricial Entropion of the Upper Lid by Tarsal Fracture.
A. Cicatricial entropion of the right upper lid. B. A horizontal incision is made
through full-thickness lid 4 mm above the lash line. Three double-armed sutures
are passed from the conjunctival surface of the attached tarsal border, between
tarsus and orbicularis of both sections of the lid, to emerge just above the lash line.
C. The sutures are tied over pegs and the lid margin everted. D. Appearance
before removal of sutures. Note good lid fold. E. Final result. Note lid margin
eversion.

line running the full length of the tarsus starting at a point lateral to the
superior punctum. Three double-armed 4-0 silk sutures, evenly spaced, are
passed through the tarsus from the conjunctival side of the superior tarsal
border then between tarsus and orbicularis to emerge on the skin surface
just above the lash line (Fig. 54B). Here the sutures are tied over pegs.

As the sutures are tied, the upper portion of the tarsus acts as a
fulcrum and the lower portion of the lid swings up with the lashes being
pulled away from the cornea (Fig. 54C). Additional skin sutures are added
for good closure (Fig. 54D). The eye is dressed daily. The tarsal sutures
should be left in 10 to 14 days to allow the tarsoconjunctival split in the lid
to granulate in well. The skin sutures are removed in 5 or 6 days. The final
result 2 months later is seen in Figure 54E.

Comment: This is a good procedure and should be used especially when other operations have failed or when entropion is extreme. Owing to the unsutured opening in the tarsoconjunctiva, granulation tissue may be overproduced and may extend below the lid margin. It can be removed by simple resection. Bringing out the sutures above the ciliary margin instead of through the lid border, as Panas did, improves the patient's comfort. The procedure is uncomplicated, the result is satisfactory, and the entropion seldom recurs.

TARSAL RESECTION WITH MUCOSAL GRAFT

In trachoma and in such conditions as pemphigus, vernal catarrh, and extensive lye burns, extreme conjunctival and tarsal cicatrization with corneal pathology often result. Corneal safety often dictates tarsal resection followed by mucous membrane grafting as the only choice.

Surgical Technic (Fig. 55): The lid is clamped and everted. An incision is made in the tarsoconjunctiva 3 mm from and following the curve of the lid border. The tarsus is dissected up from the underlying orbicularis and resected leaving a narrow rim of tarsoconjunctiva at the attached border

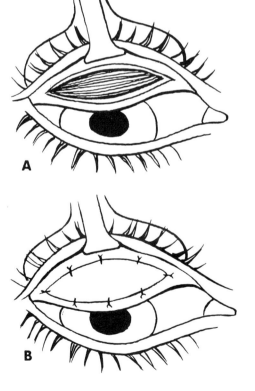

Fig. 55. Tarsal Resection with Mucosal Graft. *A.* The cicatrized tarsus is resected, leaving a 3-mm rim all around. *B.* Buccal mucous membrane fills the dehiscence. (From Fox, S. A. *Ophthalmic Plastic Surgery,* ed. 4. New York, Grune & Stratton, 1970.)

(Fig. 55A). Buccal mucosa is obtained in the usual manner and sutured into place (Fig. 55B). Thus the thickened and distorted tarsus is replaced by smooth mucous membrane, which should be cut generously to counteract the usual shrinkage.

Comment: Unless mucous membrane is grafted before closure, entropion is sure to recur owing to the loss of so much tissue from the conjunctival side of the lid. In some of the older procedures conjunctiva from the upper fornix was mobilized and drawn down to the lid border. This should not be done, as it will bring about recurrence of the entropion almost inevitably.

Dortzbach and Callahan have reported on the handling of upper lid cicatricial entropion. A novel and useful suggestion is the substitution of collagen film for an absent tarsus to provide lid rigidity (when and if necessary).

TRICHIASIS

By definition this is a clinical entity in which the lid margin remains in place but the cilia are misdirected backward impinging on the cornea and causing the patient varying degrees of discomfort. If only a few cilia are involved, they may be removed by electrolysis. But use of electrolysis should be limited because it may cause cicatrization and worse symptoms than the original trichiasis if there are many cilia to epilate.

Historically the first Z-plasty of Spencer Watson or the total marginal transplant of Dianoux has been used for severe trichiasis. Recently, a modification of the Van Millingen technic has proved effective and useful. In this technic, which is applicable to both upper and lower lid repairs, a narrow strip of tarsoconjunctiva is taken from the attached tarsal border of the ipsilateral or contralateral upper lid. The graft is planted into the split trichiatic lid border, moving the offending cilia way from the globe.

CORRECTION OF TRICHIASIS—VAN MILLINGEN'S METHOD (MODIFIED)

Surgical Technic (Fig. 56): The lid border is split in the gray line and the split deepened about 3 or 4 mm. A 3-mm strip of tarsoconjunctiva is taken from the attached tarsal border of the same or opposite upper lid. The length should be enough to fit the border split. The strip is sewn into position with interrupted sutures of 6-0 silk (Fig. 56). The tarsoconjunctival wound is closed with interrupted sutures brought out on the skin surface, as shown, where the knots will not rub against the cornea and cause the patient discomfort. Postoperative care is routine; sutures are removed on the fifth or sixth day.

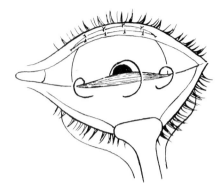

Fig. 56. Correction of Trichiasis—Van Millingen's Technic (Modified). The lid margin is split and a narrow strip of tarsoconjunctiva is resected from the attached tarsal border of the ipsilateral upper lid and planted into the lid split. The upper lid tarsoconjunctival wound is closed with interrupted silk sutures brought out and tied on *the skin surface.*

Comment: This is a modern modification of the old Van Millingen technic in which mucous membrane was used. The advantage of using tarsoconjunctiva are twofold: (1) since tarsoconjunctiva does not shrink, the exact amount can be gauged and taken, and (2) it spares the patient several days of discomfort from a sore lower lip. Although the pain from the lip wound is not prolonged and healing is relatively rapid (no lip sutures are necessary), a modification that spares the patient this discomfort is certainly worthwhile. When the graft is taken from the ipsilateral side, as is usually possible, only one eye need be patched.

An additional step which improves the procedure still more is the resection of a narrow (3-mm) horizontal strip of skin beyond the ciliary margin after the lid has been split. When the wound is sutured the ciliary margin is pulled away from the tarsoconjunctival edge and eversion is increased.

REFERENCES

Ballen, P. H. A simple procedure for the relief of trichiasis and entropion on the upper lid. *Arch. Ophthalmol.* 72:239, 1964.

Beard, C. H. *Ophthalmic Surgery,* ed. 2. Philadelphia, Blakiston, 1914, p. 253.

Burow, A. Bemerkungen zur Operation des Entropium und der Distichiasis. *Berl. Klin. Wochenschr.* 10:295, 1873.

Dalgleish, R., and Smith, J. L. S. Mechanics and history of senile entropion. *Br. Med. J.* 50:79-91, 1966.

Dianoux, E. De l'autoplastie palpébrale par le procédé de Gayet. *Ann. d'Ocul.* 2:132, 1882.

Dortzbach, R. B., and Callahan, A. Repair of cicatricial entropion of upper eyelids. *Arch. Ophthalmol.* 85:82, 1971.

Jones, L. T., Reeh, M. J., and Tsujimura, J. K. Senile entropion. *Am. J. Ophthalmol.* 55:463, 1963.

Panas, P. D'une modification apporté au procédé dit de transplantation du sol ciliare. *Arch. Ophtalmol.* 2:208, 1882.

Van Millingen, E. De la guérison radical du trichiashis par le tarso-chiloplastie. *Arch. Ophtalmol.* 8:60, 1888.

von Graefe, A. Bemerkungen zur Operation des Entropium und Ektropium. *Arch. Ophtalmol.* 10:221 (pt. 2), 1864.

Watson, T. S. On the treatment of trichiasis and distichiasis by a plastic operation. *Med. Times Gaz.* 2:546, 1874.

Wheeler, J. M. Spastic entropion correction by orbicularis transplantation. *Trans. Am. Ophthalmol. Soc.* 36:157, 1938.

Wies, F. A. Surgical treatment of entropion. *J. Int. Coll. Surg.* 21:758, 1954.

CHAPTER 7

Cosmetic Surgery

Until quite recently ophthalmic plastic surgery was mainly reparative and reconstructive. Cosmetic repairs were confined almost exclusively to the infrequent corneal tattoo or lash graft. Requirements for the former have become rare with the advent and perfection of adequately tinted contact lenses. Cilia grafting has practically disappeared for two good reasons:

    1. The results of cilia grafting are, in general, the most unsatisfactory of all ophthalmic plastic operations. Grafted cilia frequently grow too sparsely, rarely too lushly, and always irregularly, often producing trichiasis.

    2. Artificial lashes give a good cosmetic appearance and are easily applied. They are better by far than the surgeon's best efforts and are acquired at far less trouble and expense.

On the other hand, the past few years have seen an upsurge of interest by ophthalmic plastic surgeons in cosmetic lid surgery—the correction of presenile and senile lid skin atrophy (dermachalasis) and fat protrusion of the lids, and repair of the ravages of facial nerve palsies which can cause complete lagophthalmos due to upper and lower lid paralysis as well as drooping of the brow on the ipsilateral side.

This development is long overdue. Ophthalmologists have come to realize that correction of dermachalasis has gone to the general plastic surgeon by default and that the broad term "blepharoplasty"—a word of honorable and legitimate lineage—has become contracted, denigrated, and transmogrified into a colloquial expression meaning repair of lid bags.

Dermachalasis is sometimes a good deal more to the patient than a mere cosmetic blemish. Lower lids distended by too much skin and bulging with fat may cause psychologic distress of more than inconsequential proportions. Upper lids that hang so low as to impinge on the lashes may cause ocular fatigue, interfere with vision, and even become a medical problem. In our modern, youth-oriented society, a youthful appearance may be important in earning a livelihood. Hence the correction of dermachalasis is more than a purely cosmetic procedure, and it is good that ophthalmic plastic surgeons have come to realize this.

LID SKIN ATROPHY

Blepharochalasis

This is a rare condition, usually of the upper lids, most commonly appearing at puberty as an intermittent painless angioneurotic edema with redness of the lids. Over half the reported cases have been in patients under 20, with the sexes equally affected. As a result of repeated attacks loss of skin elasticity, subcutaneous atrophy, and capillary proliferation develop. The lid skin may be so stretched that it not only impinges on the lashes and interferes with vision, as in dermachalasis, but allows prolapse of orbital fat and even of the lacrimal gland. All this may happen before the patient has lived long enough to acquire the much more ordinary senile bags.

Dermachalasis: Senile Skin Atrophy

Senile or presenile lid skin atrophy should be distinguished from the more commonly named and less commonly occurring blepharochalasis described above. Baggy lids are due to slowly degenerative processes. In the younger individual they are primarily due to fat bulging through a stretched orbital fascia. In the middle aged and elderly there are usually degeneration and thinning of the skin, loss of muscle tonus, and loosening of the fibrous connections between skin and muscle or muscle and fascia orbitalis or both. Hence in older persons lid bags or puffs may consist of skin alone or, more commonly, of loose skin plus fat bulges. This is not an actual herniation of fat but a bulging through the stretched and weakened orbital fascia.

It has been shown that when orbital fat tends to work its way forward in the lids, it does so in usually predictable—and visible—areas. The

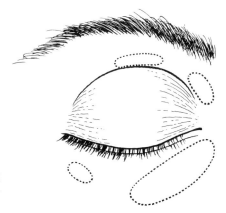

Fig. 57. Dotted Areas Indicate Usual Loci of Orbital Fat Herniation in Upper and Lower Lids.

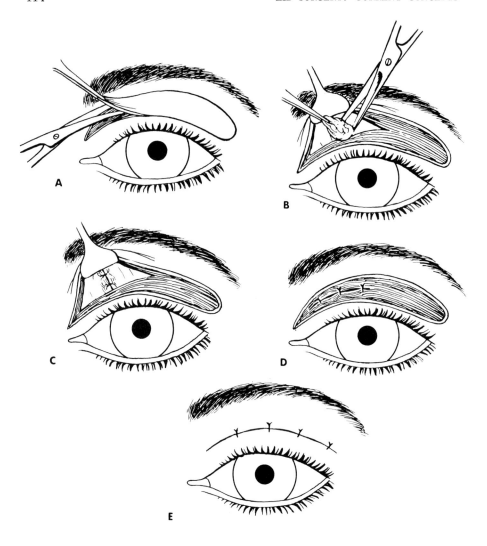

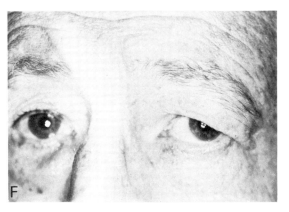

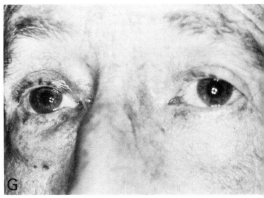

dotted areas marked out in Figure 57 show the usual, though not exclusive, loci of fat bulges in the upper and lower lids. The nasal fat bulge in the upper lid is almost always seen first; frequently it is the only one. In the lower lid also the fat bulge is usually first noted medially and this is by far the larger one; frequently two bulges are present in the lower lid, the lateral one being the smaller. Because of varying size, structure, and position, the surgical management differs for upper and lower lid skin atrophy.

CORRECTION OF UPPER LID SKIN ATROPHY—AUTHOR'S METHOD

The only treatment for both dermachalasis and blepharochalasis is surgical excision of the redundant skin and resection of prolapsed orbital fat. Both are cosmetic repairs. Man's urge to improve his appearance or correct a deformity goes back as far as history and will not be denied.

Surgical Technic (Fig. 58): The skin fold is picked up loosely and the amount to be resected marked off with an applicator dipped in sterile dye solution. The marked-off area usually tapers to a point medially, but may be rounded laterally because there is more redundant skin at the temporal side of the lid; however, the marked-off area may also come to a point laterally. It is important to mark off the area before injection swells the lid and stretches the skin. The lower line of incision should be in the lid furrow at the upper tarsal border in order to preserve a good lid fold and hide the incision scar.

The lid is then injected with a solution of 1% or 2% procaine with epinephrine 1:50,000. An Ehrhardt clamp may be inserted under the lid, which is put on slight stretch and the skin incised along the lines previously drawn. The skin is undermined and resected (Fig. 58A). The wound is closed with interrupted sutures of 6-0 braided silk placed close to the edge and the eye is patched for 24 hours (Fig. 58E). Dark glasses are then substituted, with patching optional at night. The eyes are examined and cleansed, if necessary, on the second and fourth day and the sutures are removed on the fifth day.

Resection of orbital fat is done before the skin wound is closed. Usually the fat bulges nasally. The orbicularis fibers are separated horizontally by blunt dissection, and the orbital fascia is exposed enough to permit a small vertical cut in the fascia through which the bulging fat

Fig. 58 (opposite page). Repair of Upper Lid Dermachalasis—Author's Technic. A. Lines of skin incision. Outlined skin is resected. B. In case of a fat bulge, orbicularis fibers are separated horizontally, vertical nick made in the orbital fascia, and the exposed fat is resected. C. The fascia is closed vertically (optional). D. The orbicularis fibers are closed horizontally. E. The skin wound is closed with interrupted sutures of 6-0 silk without undermining. F. Bilateral lid skin atrophy. G. Result of repair.

can prolapse and be resected (Fig. 58B). The fascia may be closed with a 6-0 chromic catgut suture (Fig. 58C) if desired. However, unless the fascial cut is very large, this suture may be omitted. With the patient lying flat the fat tends to fall back into the orbit. Hence when the patient is supine, gentle pressure should be made backward on the globe and the presenting fat resected. Unless this is done, the fat bulge will reappear when the patient is upright. The orbicularis is closed horizontally as it was opened (Fig. 58D). The skin is sutured as shown in Figure 58E. A firm supportive dressing is applied for 24 hours. A patient with upper lid dermachalasis is shown before (Fig. 58F) and after repair (Fig. 58G).

Comment: In upper lid surgery the tendency is to remove too little rather than too much skin. A good rule is to leave just enough skin so that the patient can close his eyes without tension. Taking more than this will obliterate the lid fold; taking much less will result in undercorrection.

CORRECTION OF LOWER LID SKIN ATROPHY

Dermachalasis is probably more common in the lower than in the upper lid (Fig. 59A). Lower lid bags may consist of redundant skin only or of skin plus orbital fat that has protruded through relaxed fascia. As shown in Figure 57, lower lid fat usually protrudes forward in two bundles—a larger medial clump and a smaller lateral one. Surgery to repair lower lid skin atrophy requires great care, as the lid may have to be tautened both vertically and horizontally. Since the lower lid is much narrower than the upper, overcorrection with consequent ectropion is not difficult to attain; hence circumspection must be used in skin resection.

Surgical Technic (Fig. 59): The patient is asked to look up, thus tautening lower lid skin. Whatever loose skin remains is then pinched horizontally and the amount that can be resected without causing ectropion is estimated and marked off on the lid with two parallel lines of methylene blue or gentian violet. The line of highest incision is placed close to the ciliary margin where it will be least conspicuous. The lines are carried upward for several millimeters beyond the lateral canthus following the curve of the lid. A short vertical line is then drawn downward from each end to include a small triangle (Fig. 59B). Anesthetic solution with epinephrine is injected subcutaneously. If simple skin resection is planned, it should be done cautiously—a narrow strip at a time—and the effect assessed to ensure ectropion does not result. Closure is with interrupted sutures of 5-0 or 6-0 silk (Fig. 59E).

If orbital fat is also to be resected, the skin is dissected down to the lower orbital rim, exposing the orbicularis fibers. These are carefully separated by blunt dissection in the nasal and lateral thirds, exposing the fascia with the prolapsed fat visible behind it. Two small vertical incisions are made in the fascia medially and laterally. The eye is pressed back gently into the socket and all fat that presents itself through the two openings with-

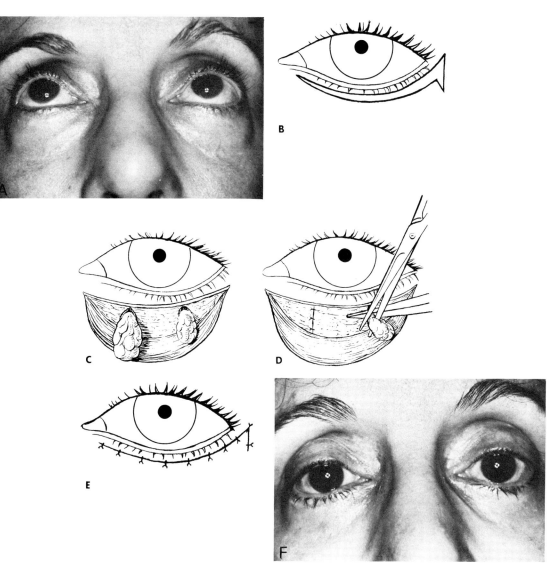

Fig. 59. Repair of Lower Lid Dermachalasis—Author's Method. *A.* Bilateral lower lid "bags." *B.* Skin incisions. *C.* Exposure of orbital fat bulges through orbital fascia. *D.* The fat is clamped and resected; the fascia is closed (optional). *E.* The skin is pulled up; excess skin is resected; and the skin is sutured. *F.* Appearance after repair.

out being pulled is resected (Fig. 59C). Hemostasis must be meticulous: The fat should be clamped before it is resected; cautery may be applied and if necessary suturing with fine catgut should be done. By whatever means, bleeding must be stopped before skin closure or discoloration may last several months. The fascia may be closed vertically with a couple of 6-0 chromic catgut sutures as in the upper lid (Fig. 59D) though this is not always necessary. The skin is closed with interrupted sutures of 6-0 silk (Fig. 59E). In closing, only enough undermining is done to bring the wound lips together snugly. The eye is patched and dressings changed every day. Sutures are removed on the fifth day, earlier if healing is good. The patch is left off in 24 or 48 hours and the patient given dark glasses to wear as protection. Figure 59F shows the final result.

Comment: It must be repeated that greater care is needed for lower lid than for upper lid dermachalasis repair. Both skin and fat should be resected cautiously. It is better to do a secondary repair for undercorrection than to risk overcorrection; replacing a bulge with ectropion or a hollow makes few friends. The orbital fascia should not be tautened too much as this also may produce ectropion. If the fascia has been opened horizontally, it should not be sutured lest ectropion develop.

Occasionally a patient complains of diplopia—usually the result of edema of the orbital tissues and consequent pressure on the bulb and ocular muscles. The diplopia will be transient unless the inferior rectus or inferior oblique muscle has been interfered with. Such muscle damage would seem impossible with the technic outlined above. One must never stick a forceps or muscle hook into the fascial opening to pull out fat. Such a maneuver can be disastrous if an inferior extraocular muscle is accidentally cut.

The lower lid may remain red and discolored for several weeks following repair unless all bleeders are well tied off and the cautery used to assure *complete* hemostasis before the skin incision is closed.

PARALYTIC LAGOPHTHALMOS

This condition is usually due to peripheral facial nerve lesions and a paralytic orbicularis. Upper lid retraction as in Graves' disease may also be a factor. A not uncommon finding is paralytic relaxation and sagging of the lid with epiphora due to inability to close the eye. Corneal damage in such cases is possible.

Repair of paralytic lagophthalmos is less a cosmetic operation than a required functional correction which incidentally makes the patient look better—a not insignificant bonus.

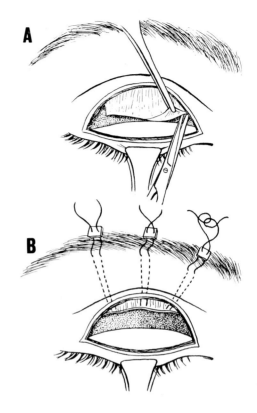

Fig. 60. Levator Recession—Author's Method. A. The levator is exposed, freed of all attachments, and allowed to retract. B. Three double-armed 4-0 silk sutures, equally spaced, are passed through the levator from behind forward. The sutures are then continued to the skin surface and tied over pegs.

REPAIR OF UPPER LID LAGOPHTHALMOS—AUTHOR'S METHOD

If the lagophthalmos is stationary and mild, some type of lateral canthoplasty (Fig. 69) will narrow the palpebral fissure, protecting the cornea and enhancing the appearance of the patient. In advanced lagophthalmos levator recession may be necessary.

Surgical Technic (Fig. 60): The levator is exposed by a transcutaneous approach as for ptosis surgery. It is freed anteriorly, posteriorly, and at the horns as for a levator resection procedure. It should now retract completely (Fig. 60A). Three equally spaced double-armed 4-0 silk sutures are passed close to the cut end of the levator from behind forward without tying. The needles are then passed anteriorly to emerge on the skin surface, where they are tied over pegs (Fig. 60B). Postoperative care is routine and the sutures are removed on the sixth day.

Comment: The amount of recession needed will depend, of course, on the degree of lagophthalmos. This can be gauged fairly accurately right on the operating table.

THE PALPEBRAL SPRING FOR REPAIR OF UPPER LID PARALYSIS

Use of the palpebral spring to correct lid paralysis was reported by Morel-Fatio and Lalardie in 1962. The spring is an ingenious little wire mechanism which passively closes the inert upper lid when the levator is relaxed. In the most recent modification of the technic the coil of the spring is anchored in the bone of the lateral orbital rim with the arms extending medially into the lid tisues. The fitting of the prosthesis is tricky. It must be done under local anesthesia since the cooperation of the patient in opening and closing the eye is necessary. Also the anesthesia must not involve the deeper tissues. Obviously this requires careful adjustment and subsequent readjustment from time to time. Not all tissues tolerate a movable metallic object without untoward reaction. Displacement or rejection of the spring due to tissue intolerance is not unknown. Nevertheless, the device has been helpful in alleviating exposure keratitis when other methods have failed.

Guy and Ransohoff report that 19 of 24 patients have been able to retain the spring with more or less comfort. There is some incompetence of the lids and complaints of dryness and a cold sensation of the cornea. However, "these are diminishing."

REPAIR OF LOWER LID LAGOPHTHALMOS

Lagophthalmos of the lower lid is associated with relaxation and sagging due to atonicity (Fig. 61A). The paralytic lower lid makes complete voluntary closure of the eye impossible. In addition the sclera below the lower limbus is exposed—a condition not calculated to enhance beauty since the difference in the position of the two lower lids is easily noticeable and often striking (Fig. 61B). Repair at both canthi is often necessary to protect the cornea (Figs. 61C and 62A) and to raise the lid. The final repair seen in figure 61D has enabled the patient to close her eye (Fig. 61E).

Repair technic varies with the condition. It may consist of bilateral canthoplasties, lateral canthoplasty and medial tarsorrhaphy, or ectropion procedures. If the lagophthalmos is of long duration ectropion may also develop; treatment then is as for paralytic ectropion.

In essence, lower lid paralytic lagophthalmos is managed much like paralytic ectropion because the two conditions are similar (identical in late stages). The only variance is that, for some reason, eversion develops late or not at all in lagophthalmos (Fig. 61A).

DROOPING OF THE BROW

In severe facial palsy the brow on the affected side may droop as well as the lower lid. To corect this Beard suggests raising the lower lid by means of medial and lateral canthoplasties as well as elevation and suture of the brow to the periosteum.

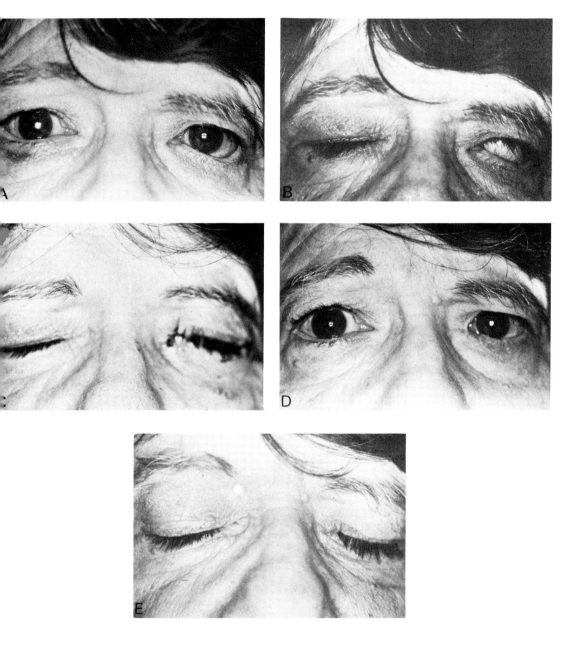

Fig. 61. Repair of Lower Lid Lagophthalmos. *A.* Lower lid paralytic lagophthalmos. *B.* Appearance on attempted closure. *C.* Repair by medial tarsorrhaphy (fig. 41) and lateral canthoplasty (fig. 62A). *D* and *E.* Appearance after
repair, with eyes open and closed.

CORRECTION OF LOWER LID AND BROW DROOP—BEARD'S METHOD

Surgical Technic (Fig. 62): The lower lid is raised by some ectropion procedure if droop is severe. If droop is of moderate degree, the lid may be raised by medial and lateral canthoplasties (Fig. 62A).

A deep incision is made just above the brow. The lower lip of the incision is undermined and the brow pulled up so that it is aligned with the contralateral normal brow. The brow is then fastened to the periosteum of the frontal bone with interrupted sutures of 4-0 chromic catgut (Fig. 62A). The frontalis muscle is closed with interrupted sutures of 4-0 plain catgut and the skin with 5-0 silk (Fig. 62B).

Comment: Skin above the brow is not excised; the excess skin is left to give some semblance of wrinkling. As Beard states, none of these procedures gives ideal results to sufferers from facial palsy, but they help— sometimes considerably.

PTOSIS OF THE LOWER LID

Blepharoptosis has always meant ptosis of the upper lid to opthalmologists; hence lower lid ptosis sounds somewhat bizarre. But ptosis does mean a

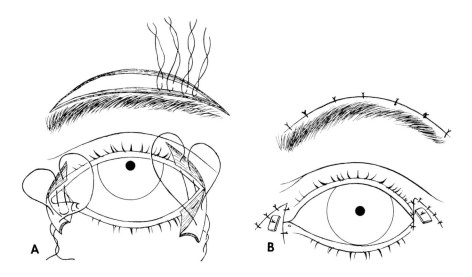

Fig. 62. Correction of Drooping of Lower Lid and Brow—Beard's Method. A. The lower lid is raised, as shown, by medial and lateral canthoplasties. An incision is made above the brow down to periosteum, the lower lip of the wound is undermined, and the drooping brow is raised and sutured to the periosteum. B. The skin wounds are closed with interrupted skin sutures.

drooping, and though lower lid drooping may be uncommon and even an oddity, it does occur. There are several types of lower lid ptosis.

1. Cicatricial ptosis is a mechanical downward displacement of the lower lid by scar, tumor, skin disease, etc. It is seen primarily in cicatricial ectropion and does not concern us here.

2. Paralytic ptosis is a downward displacement of the lower lid due to such complete atonicity that the lid sags of its own weight. The lid is so lax that it does not move up in eye closure, and sclera is exposed (Fig. 61B). Curiously the lid is rarely everted, even though the laxity is greater than in senile ectropion. Paralytic lower lid lagophthalmos has long been known and has been thoroughly described.

3. Pseudoptosis of the lower lid is seen in exophthalmos and in the higher degrees of myopia when the eyeball is proptosed beyond the normal confines of the palpebral fissure.

4. Idiopathic ptosis is a rare type characterized by a lower lid margin which rides below its normal position at the lower limbus, allowing scleral exposure although the lid is neither lengthened nor everted. The lower lid droop may be monocular (Fig. 63E) or binocular. I suspect the droop is due to relaxation of the capsulopalpebral fascia, the lower lid anlage of the levator aponeurosis. Weakness of the lower lid tarsal muscle (Müller's) may also be implicated. However, since there is no evidence of paresis or impedance of lower lid movement, I have called this type of ptosis idiopathic. It must not be confused with the lower lid downward displacement seen in proptosis and high myopia and associated with disproportionately enlarged palpebral fissures.

Idiopathic ptosis constitutes something of a cosmetic blemish especially in women of uncertain age when the bloom begins to fade a bit and facial defects become disproportionately magnified. In such cases men also are not averse to cosmetic correction especially when the blemish is emphasized by being monocular (Fig. 63E).

REPAIR OF LOWER LID PTOSIS—AUTHOR'S METHOD

The lateral canthoplasty described below was originally used for ectropion; I have found it even more useful in the repair of lower lid ptosis where punctal eversion is not a problem (Fig. 63E).

Surgical Technic (Fig. 63): The lateral quarter of the lid is split into its layers and the incision carried up beyond the canthus for an equal distance continuing the lower lid curve. From the end of this, another perpendicular and somewhat longer incision is made downward. The lid split is deepened and a triangle of tarsoconjunctiva, apex-down, is resected laterally (Fig. 63A).

The skin is undermined laterally and mobilized. It is pulled up and the excess lashes are resected from the margin (Fig. 63B, dotted line). The excess skin is also resected laterally (Fig. 63C) and the skin wound closed (Fig. 63D). Figure 63E shows the left lower lid before the operation and Figure 63F the final result.

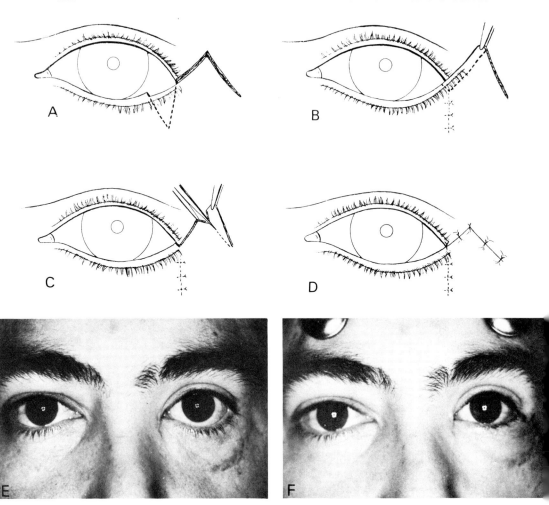

Fig. 63. Correction of Lower Lid Ptosis—Author's Technic. *A.* The lateral quarter of the lower lid is split and the split carried up and out for an equal distance following the lid curve. At the end of this incision, a perpendicular skin incision is made down and out. *B.* The resultant flap at the lateral canthus is undermined and pulled up, and the excess marginal tissue, including cilia, is resected (dotted line). *C.* Excess skin tissue is also resected laterally. *D.* The skin flap is pulled up and the wound sutured. *E.* Ptosis of left lower lid. *F.* Final result. Lower lids are now on the same level.

REFERENCES

Beard, C., Obear, M. F., Tenzel, R. R., and Smith, B. Symposium: Cosmetic blepharoplasty. *Trans. Am. Acad. Ophthalmol. Otolaryngol.* 73:1141, 1969.

Fox, S. A. A modified Kuhnt-Szymanowski procedure. *Am. J. Ophthalmol.* 62: 533, 1966.

Guy, C. L., and Ransohoff, J. The palpebral spring for paralysis of the upper eyelid. *Int. Ophthalmol. Clin.* 10:145, 1970.

Morel-Fatio, D., and Lalardie, J. P. Contributions à l'étude de la chirurgie plastique dans la paralysie facial le ressort palpébral. *Ann. Chir. Plast.* 7:275, 1962.

Morel-Fatio, D., and Lalardie, J. P. Palliative surgical treatment of facial paralysis: The palpebral spring. *Plast. Reconstr. Surg.* 33:146, 1964.

CHAPTER 8

Congenital Anomalies

Congenital anomalies continue to appear in the same old way and to take the same old forms. We now know a good deal about why they occur thanks to the tremendous strides made in genetics and related sciences. We know that chromosomal aberrations account for a large proportion of ocular genetic defects. It has been estimated that such defects are present in 1 of every 200 persons born. Although our ability in diagnosis has greatly improved, we are still unable to control or moderate the occurrence of many of these anomalies. Only some—but they are important—are of interest to the ophthalmic surgeon.

Perhaps the most important of the ophthalmic congenital anomalies are the mongoloid stigmata included in the embryonic fixation syndrome of Waardenburg (Chapter 4). This so-called "mongoloid syndrome" is a distinct genetic entity not related to the mongolism described by Langdon Down. It is inherited as an autosomal dominant, but is not associated with chromosomal abnormalities.

The patients seen by the ophthalmologist usually show relatively mild ocular abnormalities susceptible to repair but not to eradication. The common stigmata are bilateral ptosis, phimosis, and epicanthus. In addition a large proportion of patients have telecanthus—a wider than normal separation of the medial canthi.

Surgically new ways of repairing some of these long-known congenital defects are of interest. Ptosis repair and the Marcus Gunn syndrome are discussed in Chapter 4.

Epicanthus

Epicanthus is an extra fold of skin which rides over the medial canthus covering the caruncle and sometimes the plica; it thus gives the effect of shortening the palpebral fissure. It is, of course, normal in Oriental races. The epicanthus associated with the embryonic fixation syndrome is inverted: It originates in the lower, rather than the upper lid. Recently I have used two procedures to correct this condition which are quite simple and as effective as any of the more complicated technics.

CORRECTION OF EPICANTHUS—AUTHOR'S METHOD

Surgical Technic (Fig. 64): The epicanthal fold is picked up and the base on each side is incised, the two incisions meeting below the fold to form angle *a* (Fig. 64A). The resultant flap is dissected up, rotated medially, and flattened out. An incision is made along the upper border of the flap. This forms a second flap with angle *b* at the apex (Fig. 64B). This second flap is mobilized and rotated medially (Fig. 64C); the two flaps are thus transposed. They are pulled firmly into position and sutured, the needles biting into the subjacent tissues to prevent retraction (Fig. 64D).

Comment: Many of the procedures for epicanthus now in use require painstaking measurements and marking out of lines and angles before surgery. The Blair and Mustardé technics are cases in point. The distinctive feature of this flap transposition procedure is that the size and shape of the flaps depend on the proportions of each individual epicanthus and not on preconceived diagrams, sometimes quite complicated, to which the epicanthus must be fitted in Procrustean fashion. No preoperative

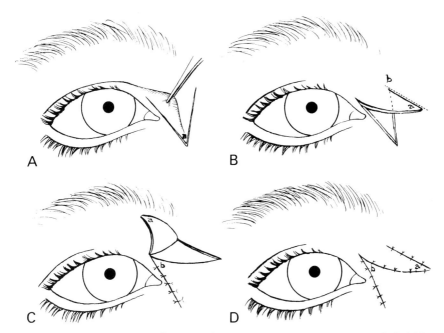

Fig. 64. Repair of Epicanthus—Author's Technic.   *A.* The epicanthal fold is raised and incised on each side, the incisions meeting at point *a*.   *B.* The resultant flap is dissected up and rotated medially; a skin incision is made along its upper border (dotted line). This forms a second flap with apex *b*.   *C.* The second flap is dissected up, mobilized, and rotated medially.   *D.* The two flaps are thus transposed and sutured into position. (From Fox, S. A. *Am. J. Ophthalmol.* 72:1144, 1971.)

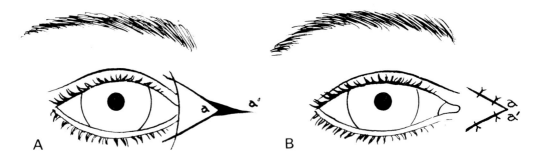

Fig. 65. Repair of Epicanthus—Verwey's Method. A. The skin is incised with a horizontal Y so that the open end of the Y straddles the epicanthus and the leg points nasally. The triangular flap (apex *a*) at the open end of the Y is raised and the lips of the incision forming the leg of the Y are undermined and separated to *a'*. B. The skin flap is pulled medially so that *a* lies at *a'*, thus converting the horizontal Y to a V and flattening out the epicanthal fold.

planning or measurement is required. There are no preliminary diagrams to mark out, no lines to measure, no angles to calculate. The surgery is simple, consisting of only three incisions; hence scarring is minimal and healing rapid. Anchorage of the flaps by deep and firm subcutaneous suture bites prevents subsequent retraction and re-formation of the epicanthus.

In epicanthus inversus, the two preliminary incisions meet at an apex *above* the epicanthal fold and the rest of the surgery is carried out accordingly.

CORRECTION OF EPICANTHUS—VERWEY'S PROCEDURE

This also is a simple procedure which in essence uses a horizontal Y-V technic.

Surgical Technic (Fig. 65): Incisions are made to form a horizontal Y with the open end straddling the epicanthus and the leg pointing nasally (Fig. 65A). The skin flap formed at the open end of the Y is dissected up, and the lips of the incision forming the leg are undermined and separated (Fig. 65A). The flap is pulled medially, converting the horizontal Y into a V and incidentally flattening out the epicanthal fold (Fig. 65B). The skin flap sutures are passed deep into the subjacent orbicularis and upper part of the medial canthal ligament to ensure firm anchorage and to reduce the tendency of the flap to retract and re-form the epicanthus. This is not unlike the Berger arrowhead technic of many years ago.

Blepharophimosis

Blepharophimosis is a reduction in size of the palpebral fissure in both dimensions. It is one of the stigmata of the embryonic fixation syndrome which requires repair. Reduction of fissure width is usually due to ptosis, discussed in Chapter 4. Lengthening of the shortened palpebral fissure is accomplished by lateral canthoplasty. Over the years three technics for lengthening the fissure have been suggested: those of von Ammon, of Agnew, and of Blair. The von Ammon procedure, the oldest (over 100 years) and simplest, has best withstood the test of time. However, they all require sectioning of the lateral canthal ligament to allow for the necessary extension. Recently Blaskovics simply resected a triangle of skin at the lateral canthus and pulled the conjunctiva out to cover the bared areas. This gives the least satisfactory result.

CORRECTION OF BLEPHAROPHIMOSIS—AUTHOR'S METHOD

The following technic for lengthening the fissure has proved effective in my hands and has been most useful.

Surgical Technic (Fig. 66): Using antiseptic dye the amount of fissure lengthening desired (usually 4 to 6 mm) is marked off from the lateral canthal angle, point *AA'*, to point *B*. The lateral quarters of the upper and lower lids are split close to the posterior edge, and the whole area included in the broken line arc is undermined. The dissection is not carried beyond *B* since this is a fixed point. The incision in the upper lid margin is prolonged downward about 4 mm following the upper lid curve to point *C*, then to *B* (Fig. 66A).

The flap *ACB* is allowed to retract so that *C* comes to rest at or close to *A* and the points are sutured skin-to-skin (Fig. 66B). The lower flap (apex *A'*) is mobilized, drawn out to *B*, and sutured. Thus the new skin canthus is formed as shown by its extension beyond the broken vertical line from its orginal position (Fig. 66C).

The conjunctiva is grasped at its lateral point and carefully undermined medially as much as necessary (Fig. 66D). It is drawn laterally as far as its elasticity will allow and sutured to the upper and lower edges of the cut skin and at *B*. A double-armed suture is passed through the conjunctiva at the new canthal angle and brought out on the skin surface beyond the canthus, where it is tied over a peg (Fig. 66E). This will help deepen the new canthal angle and keep it from flattening out and gaping. The eye is patched and dressed daily; the sutures are removed on the fifth or sixth day.

Comment: Although well over 100 years old, the von Ammon procedure is still the most commonly used because it is the simplest. However, it is frequently inadequate because the tissues are not mobilized

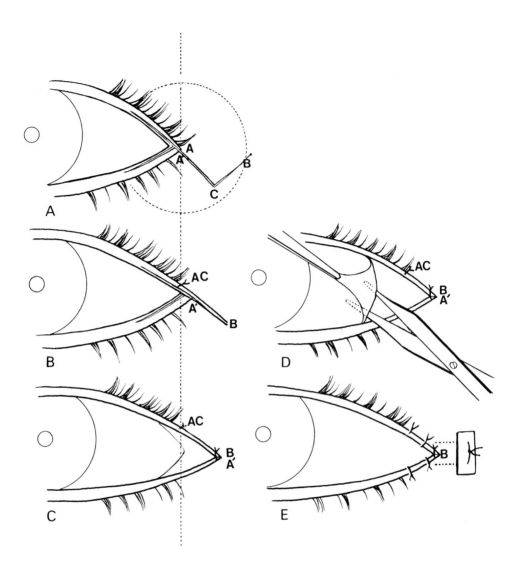

Fig. 66. Correction of Blepharophimosis—Author's Technic. A. The amount of fissure lengthening desired is marked off from the canthal angle, point *AA'*, to point *B*. The lateral quarters of the upper and lower lids are split, and the whole area included in the broken line arc is undermined. The incision in the upper lid margin is extended down about 4 mm to *C*, then to *B*. B. The flap *ACB* is mobilized and allowed to retract. Point *C* is sutured at *A*. C. The lower flap is mobilized, pulled laterally, and *A'* is sutured at *B*. D. The conjunctiva is under-mined and separated from its bed. E. The conjunctiva is pulled out and sutured to the edges of the new skin canthus. A double-armed suture is passed under the new lateral canthal angle to deepen it and prevent gaping. (From Fox, S. A. *Arch. Ophthalmol.* 86:407, 1971.)

sufficiently. An unsightly gaping sometimes occurs at the new canthal angle because the conjunctiva has been pulled out beyond its elastic limit.

The procedure outlined above provides the lengthening required, as both skin and conjunctiva are well mobilized. Since the lateral canthal ligament is not cut, the foundation of the new canthal angle will not tend to be displaced. Also the freed conjunctiva is left intact and is simply pulled out to the extent of its normal elasticity and no further.

Since not all lids are alike the amount of required undermining varies; the flaps may have to be trimmed or lengthened a little for good closure. The above procedure provides cosmetically acceptable 5 to 6 mm lengthening of the palpebral fissure.

Telecanthus

Telecanthus, a widening of the medial intercanthal distance, is another of the congenital defects commonly associated with the embryonic fixation syndrome. One repair method proposed involves wiring together the two medial canthal ligaments through the nose, thus drawing the canthi together. Since the success of this maneuver depends on the elasticity and extensibility of the canthal ligaments and attached tissues and not on the tensile strength of the wires uniting them, it would seem that correction could be more easily and simply accomplished by a forceful shortening of each ligament by either tucking or resection. A couple of stout silk sutures only would be needed, which could be left buried.

CORRECTION OF TELECANTHUS

Surgical Technic (Fig. 67): The medial canthal ligament is exposed as for a sac operation. Once the ligament is in view, a stout white silk or linen suture is passed close to the bony attachment of the ligament. The needle is then passed through the ligament again about 5 or 6 mm more laterally. The suture is tied and the ligament thus tucked and pulled nasally. If too large a bite is taken, it will not be possible to effect a complete tuck, as the ligament has only so much "give," especially in the

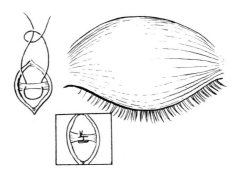

Fig. 67. Tucking of Medial Canthal Ligament. A stout white linen suture is used to create a tuck (*inset*).

young. However, a shortening of 3 to 4 mm is usually possible. When tucking is done bilaterally a wide medial intercanthal space may be appreciably narrowed.

Comment: This procedure is usually done in conjunction with a lateral cantholysis which allows the lids to be pulled medially and hence facilitates the procedure.

Epiblepharon

This condition is a developmental anomaly in which an accessory fold of skin runs horizontally close to the ciliary margin of the upper (epiblepharon superior) or, more commonly, lower (epiblepharon inferior) eyelid.

It is a congenital deformity in Caucasians, rare in the upper lid but more common in the lower lid. With the exception of blepharoptosis, epiblepharon is probably the most common congenital abnormality seen by the ophthalmologist. The patients are usually less than a year old and are brought in because of corneal irritation of varying severity.

The surgical importance of epiblepharon inheres in the fact that the accessory skin fold sometimes pushes the lashes and even the lid margin against the globe, with consequent secondary entropion and severe irritation of the conjunctiva and cornea. (Epiblepharon should not be confused with congenital entropion, in which the *whole margin* of the lid is turned in without the obvious presence of an accessory skin fold.) Rarely both congenital entropion and congenital epiblepharon are present. Both are cured simultaneously by the procedure described below.

Since epiblepharon is sometimes not sufficiently severe to require surgery and the skin fold tends to involute and disappear by the end of the first year or even somewhat later, surgical intervention should not be precipitate. On the other hand, I have seen severely inflamed eyes and cloudy corneas in a 4-month-old baby who was obviously in great distress and needed surgical succor.

CORRECTION OF EPIBLEPHARON—AUTHOR'S METHOD

This condition lends itself easily to repair by the resection of a horizontal strip of skin and some orbicularis muscle fibers.

Surgical Technic (Fig. 68): The excess skin is pinched up and marked off with an antiseptic dye. The skin is resected along with some fibers of the subjacent orbicularis (Fig. 68A). On closure the lashes should be rotated outward and pointing away from the globe (Fig. 68B). If not, another narrow strip of skin is resected. I prefer to use this conservative method. Undercorrection is simply handled; overcorrection is a complication I prefer to be spared.

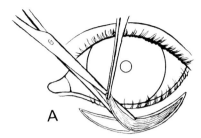 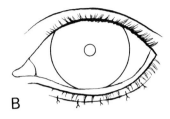

Fig. 68. Repair of Epiblepharon—Author's Technic. *A.* Horizontal strips of skin and muscle are resected. *B.* Closure is made with the lashes now pointing away from the globe.

Euryblepharon

Euryblepharon (*eurus,* broad; *blepharon,* lid) is a congenital anomaly in which the lids are enlarged and both dimensions of the palpebral fissure are symmetrically lengthened. There are usually lateral displacement of the lateral canthi and some lateral ectropion. Repair includes some type of lateral canthoplasty to shorten the palpebral fissure. Figure 69 shows the pre- and postoperative appearance of a patient with euryblepharon. Repair was accomplished by full-thickness lid wedge resection and Fuchs' lateral canthoplasty (Fig. 70).

SHORTENING THE PALPEBRAL FISSURE—FUCHS' METHOD (MODIFIED)

There are several good canthoplasties for shortening the palpebral fissure. Over the years the Fuchs technic has been the most effective and popular. However, one disadvantage is the tendency for the lids to separate at the medial end of the skin-muscle union and thus negate some of the shortening. In the past few years I have found the following modification most effective in keeping the lids from separating.

Surgical Technic (Fig. 70): The lids are brought together and the amount of shortening required is marked off on both lids by a vertical scratch or a line of antiseptic dye. An incision is made along the line through skin and muscle and then laterally along the gray line of each lid to the external angle. The resultant triangular flaps are undermined and the upper one is resected as is the ciliary margin of the lower one (Fig. 70A). The marginal epithelium of the bared tarsoconjunctiva of both lids is shaved off and the edges firmly sutured together with 4-0 chromic catgut (Fig. 70B). The lower skin-muscle flap is pulled up and sutured into the bared area of the opposing lid (Fig. 70C).

Comment: Suturing of the tarsoconjunctival edges strengthens the line of fusion and helps retain the planned amount of fissure shortening.

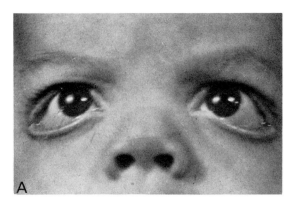 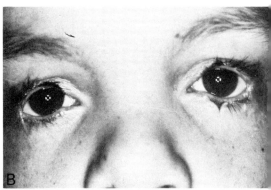

Fig. 69. Repair of Euryblepharon. A. Preoperative appearance. B. The lids and fissure have been shortened. See text.

The technic is reversible: if necessary the skin-muscle flap from the lower lid may be resected and the upper lid flap pulled down and sutured into the lower lid after the tarsoconjunctiva is fused.

Congenital Ectropion

This unusual condition is rarely seen by the opthalmologist as a primary disorder. It may occur secondarily in microphthalmos, buphthalmos, and euryblepharon or, even more rarely, combined with epicanthus and phimosis. Surgery might well be postponed because the sparse reports of this condition indicate that there is a spontaneous reinversion of the ectropion in the rare cases when it appears alone.

Congenital Entropion

Unlike senile entropion the congenital type is due to hypertrophy of the marginal orbicularis fibers; deficiency of the tarsal plate has also been reported. The lower lid is most often affected. However, Hiles and Wilder have recently reported a patient with congenital bilateral upper lid entropion. Correction is relatively easily accomplished in both upper and lower lids by resection of a horizontal spindle of skin and muscle, as for epiblepharon (Fig. 68). Surgery should be conservative, lest the entropion be converted to ectropion.

Distichiasis

Distichiasis is a double row of marginal lashes consisting of the normal anterior margin cilia and an accessory posterior row of lashes emerging from the openings of the area usually occupied by the meibomian glands. In primitive animals the meibomian glands are known to be modified sebaceous glands having lashes; presumably the lashes have disappeared during man's evolution. Hence embryologically, distichiasis may be a simple heterotypical differentiation in which the meibomian glands are replaced by cilia (Duke-Elder). The condition has been known and reported for at least 150 years.

Distichiasis occurs, though rarely, as an inherited familial trait along with other anomalies. Deutsch has reported eight members of three generations of a family with congenital distichiasis and epicanthus. The mode of inheritance was autosomal and dominant. Since distichiasis has also been known to appear in older individuals, it can probably be acquired as a result of long-standing inflammations of the lid such as Stevens-Johnson disease.

The ophthalmologic importance of distichiasis lies in the irritation of the cornea by the accessory lashes. The extra lashes may be few and occur on only one or two lids or they may be profuse and be found on all four lids. Since the lashes are usually small, soft, practically colorless, and often quite sparse, they are sometimes tolerated better than might be expected. However, if the extra lashes have all the characteristics of normal cilia, they can produce severe ocular irritation and should be removed.

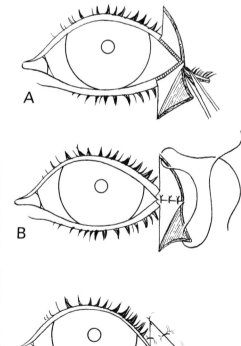

Fig. 70. Shortening of the Palpebral Fissure—Fuchs' Method (Modified). *A.* The amount of fissure shortening is estimated, the skin-muscle flaps are outlined, and the upper one is resected. The cilia are resected from the lower flap. *B.* The marginal epithelium of the bared tarsoconjunctival edges of both flaps is shaved off and the edges sutured together firmly. *C.* The lower skin-muscle flap is pulled up and sutured into the bared area of the upper lid. (From Fox, S. A. *Arch. Ophthalmol.* 86:407, 1971.)

When the supernumerary lashes are few, epilation—manually or by electrolysis—may suffice. However, if more then four or five lashes are present, electrolysis may cause cicatrization and more definitive surgical treatment is necessary. This takes two forms: (1) a marginal graft of mucous membrane for mild distichiasis and (2) resection of the tarsoconjunctiva containing the offending lashes, followed by plastic repair, for severe distichiasis.

LASH RESECTION AND MARGINAL MUCOUS MEMBRANE GRAFT

Surgical Technic (Fig. 71): The lid is split in the gray line and the incision deepened sufficiently to permit resection of the offending posterior row of lashes with their root bulbs (Fig. 71A). A narrow strip of mucous membrane is obtained from the patient's lower lip and fastened into position with a few 6-0 silk retaining sutures to replace the resected posterior margin (Fig. 71B). Postoperative care is routine and the sutures should be removed on the fifth day.

Comment: The mucous membrane tends to shrink; hence the graft should be cut generously. The procedure for taking mucous membrane has been reported elsewhere and will not be repeated here. A recent modification—and a good one—is the use of a narrow strip of tarsoconjunctiva from the attached border of the ipsilateral upper lid instead of mucous membrane. This is discussed in connection with the repair of trichiasis (Chapter 6 and Fig. 56).

LASH RESECTION AND PLASTIC REPAIR
In severe distichiasis with many more lashes present (Fig. 72A), a more definitive type of surgery is necessary.

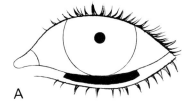

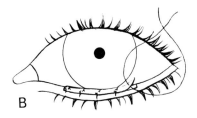

Fig. 71. Correction of Distichiasis by Mucous Membrane or Tarsoconjunctival Graft. A. The tarsoconjunctival flap is mobilized and the portion containing the offending adventitious cilia is resected. B. A strip of mucous membrane or tarsoconjunctiva fills in the marginal tarsoconjunctival dehiscence.

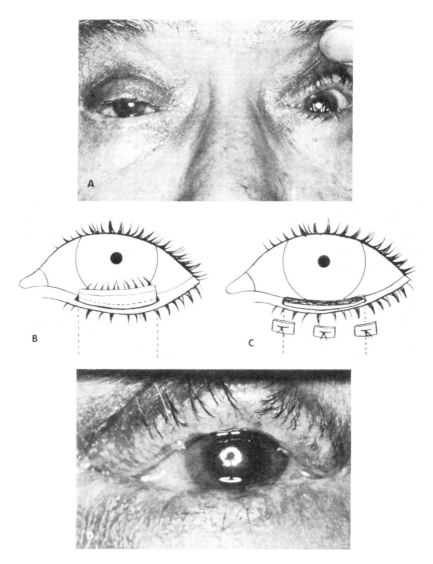

Fig. 72. Correction of Distichiasis by Resection and Plastic Repair—Author's Technic. *A.* Distichiasis of the left lower lid. Note the accessory row of lashes against the cornea. *B.* The lid is split in the gray line. A sliding tarsoconjunctival flap is mobilized by means of two lateral incisions, pulled up, and the offending lashes resected. *C.* The tarsoconjunctival lamina is pulled up slightly above the skin-muscle lamina and sutured into position with three double-armed 4-0 silk sutures passed through both laminae from behind forward and tied over pegs. The two lateral sutures straddle the verticle tarsoconjunctival incision. *D.* Final result. (From Fox, S. A. *Ophthalmic Plastic Surgery,* ed. 4. New York, Grune & Stratton, 1970.)

Surgical Technic (Fig. 72): After suitable instillation and infiltration anesthesia, the lid is split and the dissection carried downward to attain complete separation of the two laminae. A vertical incision is made through the tarsoconjunctival lamina close to each canthus (Fig. 72B, dotted lines) thus creating a sliding flap of tarsoconjunctiva. The upper 3 mm of this flap containing the offending accessory cilia is resected (Fig. 72B, horizontal dotted line). When the flap is completely mobile, it is pulled up so that its cut edge slightly overrides the anterior skin-muscle edge to counteract subsequent retraction, and the two vertical conjunctival incisions are closed with interrupted sutures of 6-0 chromic catgut.

Three double-armed 4-0 silk sutures are passed through both laminae from the conjunctival surface forward about 2 mm below the margin and tied over a peg. One of these double-armed sutures is centrally placed. Each of the side sutures is so located as to straddle the medial and lateral incisions in the tarsoconjunctiva (Fig. 72C).

A firm dressing is applied and changed at 2-day intervals. Sutures are removed on the tenth day. The final result is shown in Figure 72D.

Comment: In a patient with Stevens-Johnson disease seen by the author both upper and lower lids were involved. Tarsoconjunctival sliding grafts were fashioned in both lids and the repair carried out according to the above technic except that raw tarsoconjunctival edges of the upper and lower lids were sutured to each other and separated later, on healing. This worked quite well.

Overcorrection by pulling the tarsoconjunctival flap beyond the skin-muscle lamina is important to allow for retraction and to counteract the lid's tendency to become entropic because of the loss of tarsoconjunctiva. If entropion does occur, a von Graefe procedure (Fig. 53) restores the balance.

REFERENCES

Agnew, C. R. *Cantho-Plasty as a Remedy in Certain Diseases of the Eye.* New York, Putnam, 1875.

von Ammon, F. *Klinische Darstellingen der angeborenen Krankheiten des Auges und der Augenlider.* Berlin, Reimer, 1841.

Berger, E. Epicanthus. *Arch. Ophtalmol.* 18:453, 1898.

Blair, V. P. Lateral canthoplasty. *Am. J. Ophthalmol.* 15:498–503, 1932.

Blaskovics, L. Cited by H. Arruga. *Ocular Surgery.* New York, McGraw-Hill, 1953.

Deutsch, A. R. Distichiasis and epicanthus. *Ann. Ophthalmol.* 3:168, 1971.

Duke-Elder, S. *System of Ophthalmology.* St. Louis, Mosby, vol. 3, pt. 2, 1963, p. 873.

Feric-Seiwerth, F., Celić, M., and Domljan, Z. Marcus Gunn syndrome. *Klin. Monatsbl. Augenheilkde.* 154:519, 1969.

Fox, S. A. Primary congenital entropion. *Arch. Ophthalmol.* 56:839–842, 1956.

Fox, S. A. Distichiasis. *Am. J. Ophthalmol.* 53:14, 1962.

Fox, S. A. Lengthening and shortening the palpebral fissure. *Arch. Ophthalmol.* 86:407, 1971.

Fox, S. A. Simple epicanthus procedure. *Am. J. Ophthalmol.* 72:1144, 1971.

Fuchs, E., *Textbook of Ophthalmology,* ed.2 New York, Appleton, 1905, p. 798.

Goodman, R. M., and Gorlin, R. J. *The Face in Genetic Disorders.* St. Louis, Mosby, 1970, p. 58.

Hiles, D. A., and Wilder, L. W. Congenital entropion of the upper lids. *J. Pediatr. Ophthalmol.* 6:157, 1969.

Iliff, C. E. The optimum time for surgery in the Marcus Gunn phenomenon. *Trans. Am. Acad. Ophthalmol. Otolaryngol.* 74:1005, 1970.

Mustardé, J. C. Epicanthal folds and problem of telecanthus. *Trans. Ophthalmol. Soc. U.K.* 83:397, 1963.

Verwey, A., Over het maskergelaat en zijn behandeling. *Net. tij. v. gen.* 45:1596, 1909.

Waardenburg, P. J., Franceschetti, A., and Klein, D. *Genetics in Ophthalmology,* vol. 1. Oxford, Blackwell Scientific Publications, 1961, p. 415.

Lacrimal Disorders

Tearing is a problem, sometimes a challenge, frequently a headache—not always in that order. It is a problem which may be easily solved; on the other hand, it may offer a challenge which is a headache indeed. This has been so for a long time, and the past few years have not brought forth much new information to comfort the embattled ophthalmologist or the distressed patient.

On the basis of anatomic findings, Brienen and Snell have concluded that the principal—the only—force that drives the tears from the conjunctival sac into the nasolacrimal duct is the positive pressure generated in the sac by orbicularis contraction (and lid closure). The sac and canaliculi play no part. This conclusion would seem to be borne out by the adequate drainage established after punctal snipping (whether one or more snips) and after conjunctivodacryocystorhinostomy (CDCR). This knowledge is of no great help, however, in curing lacrimal obstruction.

EPIPHORA IN INFANTS

To this day some pediatricians still advise parents of children with tearing disorders to wait, assuring them that the condition "will clear up by itself." Frequently the ophthalmologist is consulted too late for any but drastic measures, as pointed out by Murecki and by Kohler and Muller. The latter reported 99 successful probings out of 100 for lacrimal stenosis in infants under 1 year. (They probed and irrigated through the upper canaliculus.) However, older children required dacryocystorhinostomy (DCR). Murecki points out that the rate of successful intranasal DCR in children diminishes with the increased age of the child. He attributes this to congenital defects and increased formation of granulation tissue. In fact, his results were better in adults than in older children.

Some way must be found to alert all pediatricians to the importance of submitting children with tearing problems for treatment at the earliest possible moment. The first few weeks of life are the best. The success rate diminishes with every month the infant ages. Treatment of these infants is so well standardized as to require no repetition here. What is required is increased and early cooperation from pediatricians.

EPIPHORA IN ADULTS

Nasolacrimal Duct Obstruction

Excluding emotional stimulation or surface irritation the most common cause of tearing in adults is obstruction of the nasolacrimal duct. Probing and dacryocystectomy had their heyday several decades ago. Modern ophthalmic surgeons have found the DCR more effective. This is now the operation of choice and justly so.

ILIFF'S DCR PROCEDURE

Iliff has recently reported an improved version of his successful DCR procedure.

Surgical Technic (Fig. 73): After making the opening into the sac and nasal mucosa he does not suture them together, but passes the tip of a French No. 14 urethral catheter into the nose (Fig. 73A). The proximal end is resected and is fastened inside the neck of the sac with a 3-0 chromic catgut suture. The distal end is fastened to the ala of the nose (Fig. 73B).

Comment: Iliff reports 87 such operations with an overall success rate of 90 per cent. His report should be read in its entirety.

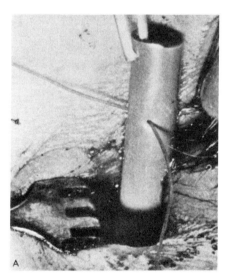 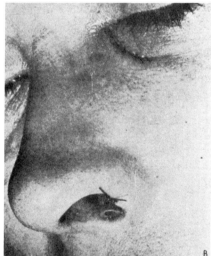

Fig. 73. Dacryocystorhinostomy—Iliff's Method. A. The proximal end of a catheter is pulled into the neck of the lacrimal sac. B. The distal end of the catheter is sutured at the exteral naris.

Pico has reported a series of 121 patients treated by DCR with only 4 failures and 1 serious complication. His technic includes a skin incision 3 mm from the canthus and cutting the medial canthal ligament to obtain good exposure. Two important modifications are (1) passing a suture from the punctum down into the nares, the suture being left in place and moved at every dressing to dislodge inspissated hemorrhage and debris which might obstruct the nasal passages; and (2) suturing only the posterior flap of the sac to the nasal mucosa; the anterior flap is sutured to the nasal periosteum. Pico's technic is meticulous, which may account at least in part for his excellent results.

Tenzel reports good results in obstructions of the common punctum by doing a DCR and reopening the common punctum by simple resection of obstructing tissue.

Krasnov reports a new use for ultrasonography in 41 cases. He uses the instrument for resecting bone to fashion the nasal window for the DCR operation. Apparently this is a safe and simple procedure—and a remarkable innovation. However, nothing should surprise us these days. Repetition and confirmation by other surgeons should simplify the DCR procedure considerably.

Canalicular Obstruction

This is a much more stubborn condition than nasolacrimal obstruction, but fortunately more rare. For correction, regardless of cause, the CDCR is the accepted procedure. Two types of tubes are now in use: The Jones Pyrex tube and the Reinecke and Carroll Silastic elbow tube. Both are valuable and I have had good results with both. Insertion of the Silastic tube is a simple procedure which does not require a secondary Pyrex tube installation, as is the case with the Jones tube. I have left Reinecke and Carroll tubes in for 3 years without the least untoward symptoms. Plans to fashion the tube of hydrophilic material should make it even more acceptable.

Henderson has suggested a simplified procedure for the insertion of the polyethylene tube in CDCR operations. He uses a guide wire and trephine to make a passage into the sac. The same wire left in place facilitates insertion of the polyethylene tube.

The simplest operation is a conjunctivorhinostomy reported by Raine which can be done as an office or outpatient procedure under local anesthesia: After resection of the caruncle, a 2.5-mm Steinman pin is used to drill a hole from the conjunctival sac to a point beneath the middle turbinate. A Jones Pyrex tube is immediately inserted after hemostasis.

The procedure has been used in 52 patients with a success rate of about 80 per cent. Apparently few postoperative problems have been encountered over the 2.5 years the technic has been in use.

Cox has devised a set of graduated Pyrex tubes for the CDCR opera-

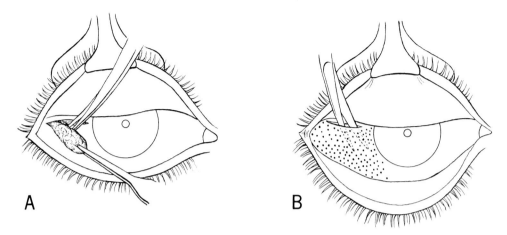

Fig. 74. Combined Resection of Palpebral Lacrimal Gland and Section of Lacrimal Ductules to Relieve Epiphora—Author's Technic. *A.* The lateral conjunctiva is incised at the upper tarsal border and the palpebral lobe of the lacrimal gland resected. *B.* The medial conjunctiva is undermined down to the lower tarsus.

tion to accommodate the anatomic variations of patients. With the set comes a precision millimeter gauge for determining the proper length of the tube and a steel rod with Teflon inserter to facilitate placement of the tube.

These rapidly multiplying improvements to simplify the DCR and CDCR operations would seem to leave little except computer surgery as the next step. Not quite yet though.

RESECTION OF PALPEBRAL GLAND PLUS JAMESON SECTION OF LACRIMAL DUCTULES—AUTHOR'S MODIFICATION

The problem of epiphora is too vast to be covered in a small specialized book such as this. Furthermore it is a problem which has been repeatedly discussed in recent ophthalmic literature. Strangely enough, however, the procedure I have found quite useful lately is an old operation, or rather, a fusion of two old operations which according to my recent experience, has been undeservedly neglected. It is a resection of the palpebral portion of the lacrimal gland combined with a section of the lacrimal ductules as described by Jameson years ago. This combination does not always cure the tearing, but it almost always ameliorates it sufficiently to relieve the patient of the worst symptoms. Hence it is worth trying. I have never seen a dry eye as the result of this operation—or an eye in which tearing has been reduced below the normal level. The technic is quite simple.

Surgical Technic (Fig. 74): Anesthesia is obtained by conjunctival instillation of 0.5% tetracaine and infiltration of the lateral half of the conjunctival sac with 1% procaine or lidocaine with epinephrine. The area is massaged until the anesthesia is well absorbed.

The upper lid is everted on an Ehrhardt clamp and the eye rotated down and in. The accessory lobe of the gland usually presents immediately as a bulge beneath the conjunctiva just below the outer edge of the tarsus. If not, a blunt instrument pressing behind the everted lid brings it into view.

An incision is made in the conjunctiva along the attached tarsal border from the outer canthus to the upper corneal limbus (Fig. 74A). As the conjunctiva is undermined the palpebral lobe of the lacrimal gland comes into view, and the conjunctiva is dissected away from its capsule. The gland is grasped and carefully resected from its surroundings without injury to the levator or fascia. The palpebral portion of the lacrimal gland is a lobulated structure and varies in size and consistency. It may be large and compact or may consist of many small discrete lobules. In any case the dissection can be easily accomplished (Fig. 74A).

After the gland lobules are excised, the lips of the conjunctival wound are spread and the conjunctiva is undermined to include the whole lateral half of the conjunctival sac. By this means all the openings of the lacrimal ductules are sectioned, including those that lie in the lower lateral fornix (Fig. 74B).

The wound is re-examined to make sure that no remnants of the gland are left behind and closed with a few 6-0 chromic catgut sutures. The conjunctival sac is irrigated and a firm pressure dressing applied for 48 hours. The eye will remain injected for a couple of weeks.

Comment: It has been stated that removal of the entire palpebral lobe of the lacrimal gland destroys the two to six main secretory ductules from the main lobe and hence the entire secretory function of both lobes is inactivated. Nothing of the sort happens. As a matter of fact, in earlier days, when dacryocystectomy was a favorite operation, Wheeler advised removal of the palpebral lacrimal gland at the same time to diminish tearing. The main postoperative complication I have noted is that tearing is not always sufficiently reduced.

Neither section of the lacrimal ductules by itself, as suggested by Jameson, nor extirpation of the palpebral portion of the lacrimal gland will cause complete cessation of lacrimation. However, the combined operation is usually effective in reducing tearing to bearable proportions, which is a relief to the patient. Jameson's instructions call for the conjunctival incision to be made *below* the external commissure. However, in the combined operation it is simpler to use the higher up incision as described above in order to undermine the conjunctiva. The dissection should be just beneath the conjunctiva so that the points of the scissors are always visible. In this way injury to the levator or the fascia with release of orbital fat will be avoided. The surgery is simple and the healing prompt although the conjunctiva may remain injected for some time. Jameson originally used no closing sutures. However, there seems to be nothing gained from leaving the wound open; sutures hasten healing.

For some reason, it takes several weeks—sometimes 5 or 6—before the full effect is obtained and the patient is disappointed at first. Then one fine day, after what seems a long time after operation, the patient will gleefully announce that the tearing has stopped or has diminished considerably.

Compared with a DCR or a CDCR, with its always potentially troublesome emplaced tube, the procedure described above is so simple that it seems worth trying in all cases of lacrimal duct obstruction before the nasal bone is punctured and mucous membrane messed up.

ACUTE DACRYOCYSTITIS

Lebensohn has called attention to an excellent old technic, first suggested by Agnew, for emptying the acutely infected lacrimal sac. This procedure was exhumed and reported by Verhoeff some 60 years ago but it never attained the popularity it deserves. Only when one realizes that Agnew devised this procedure in an era when leeches and hot poultice were the treatments of choice does one begin to appreciate the intellectual acumen of great ophthalmologists of earlier days.

SURGICAL TREATMENT OF ACUTE DACRYOCYSTITIS—AGNEW'S PROCEDURE

Surgical Technic (Fig. 75): An angular keratome is inserted just in front of the caruncle, then plunged into the sac to the bone; the incision is enlarged by cutting upward and outward. The lacrimal duct is immediately probed through the incision with a large probe. The probing is repeated on alternate days to keep the wound open and the patient is instructed to press on the sac from time to time to empty it and to keep the palpebral fissure free of pus by frequent irrigations. In most cases the cure is complete in a week.

Comment: Verhoeff pointed out that this incision involved cutting through the least possible depth of tissue and ensured constant irrigation of

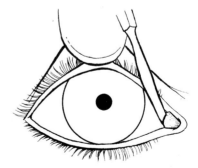

Fig. 75. Relief of Acute Dacryocystitis—Agnew's Method. A keratome is entered anterior to the caruncle and pushed to the nasal bone; the incision is enlarged upward and outward. This is followed by probing.

the lacrimal sac by the tears. His objection to the skin incision was that, owing to the depth of the wound, drainage was imperfect, frequently requiring a drain which in turn might cause a fistula. This is an excellent technic which like Jameson's section of the lacrimal ductules has long been buried in obscurity. It deserves a better fate as, probably, do many others. For to paraphrase the poet:

> Full many a surgical gem of purest ray serene
> The dark forgotten literature does bear,
> And many technics are born to blush unseen
> And waste their virtue on the desert air.
>   *Derivative doggerel by Fox*

THE SICCA SYNDROME AND KERATOPATHY

The dry eye can be even more troublesome than the wet one because the cornea and vision itself may be ultimately compromised. Work continues in diagnosis and therapy but there are few new developments in surgery. Punctal cautery and canthoplasties continue to be the surgical mainstays, but at best surgical treatment is not trustworthy in this condition. However, the subject is far too important to be ignored completely, even in this book.

Bysterfeld has shown that the lysozyme test for keratitis sicca is by far the most reliable diagnostic tool; where Schirmer's test can be wrong in 16 per cent of cases, the lysozyme test fails in only 1 per cent. It is done by testing the affect of tear lysozyme on a meat-infusion agar plate incubated for 24 hours at 36° C.

Gould feels that one of the most effective treatments of the dry eye is the fitting of a scleral contact lens. Dramatic results are obtained in patients with chronic Stevens-Johnson syndrome: Within several days corneal moisture is restored and maintained for several years. Patients with keratoconjunctivitis sicca also improved. Exposure keratitis and ocular pemphigus were harder to treat. However, an overall good response of over 75 per cent can be expected.

The use of Griffin hydrophilic contact lenses as corneal bandages has been reported by Gasset and Kaufman. They have had gratifying results in the treatment of keratitis sicca, bullous keratopathy, ocular pemphigus, and Stevens-Johnson disease. Buxton and Locke reported hydrophilic lenses gave good results in the treatment of corneal ulcers and dry eyes, but were less successful in the treatment of advanced bullous keratopathy.

REFERENCES

Brienen, J. A., and Snell, C.A.R.D. The mechanism of lacrimal flow. *Ophthalmologica* 159:223, 1969.

Bysterfeld, O. P. Diagnostic tests in the sicca syndrome. *Arch. Ophthalmol.* 82:10, 1969.

Buxton, J. N., and Locke, C. R. Evaluation of hydrophilic lenses. *Am. J. Ophthalmol.* 72:532, 1971.

Cox, C. W. Mechanical adjunct for lacrimal drainage. *Am. J. Ophthalmol.* 72:931, 1971.

Gasset, A. R., and Kaufman, H. E. Hydrophilic lens. *Am. J. Ophthalmol.* 71:1185, 1971.

Gould, H. L. The dry eye and scleral contact lenses. *Am. J. Ophthalmol.* 70:37, 1970.

Henderson, P. N. A trephining technic for the insertion of the Lester Jones tube. *Arch. Ophthalmol.* 85:448, 1971.

Iliff, C. E. A simplified DCR. *Arch. Ophthalmol.* 85:586, 1971.

Jameson, P. C. Subconjunctival section of the ductules of the lacrimal gland as a cure for epiphora. *Arch. Ophthalmol.* 17:207, 1937.

Kohler, V., and Muller, W. The treatment of stenosis of the lacrimal passages in infants. *Ophthalmolgica* 159:136, 1969.

Krasnov, M. M. Ultrasonic dacryocystorhinostomy. *Am. J. Ophthalmol.* 72:200, 1971.

Murecki, R. Intubation of lacrimal canaliculi in children. *J. Pediatr. Ophthalmol.* 7:174, 1970.

Murecki, R. Late results after intranasal dacryocystorhinostomy in infants. *J. Pediatr. Ophthalmol.* 8:38, 1971.

Pico, G. A modified technique of external dacryocystorhinostomy. *Am. J. Ophthalmol.* 72:679, 1971.

Raine, A. C. Office conjunctivorhinostomy. *Ann. Ophthalmol.* 3:1097, 1971.

Reinecke, R. D., and Carroll, J. M. Silicone lacrimal tube implantation. *Trans. Am. Acad. Ophthalmol. Otolaryngol.* 73:85, 1969.

Tenzel, R. R. Canaliculodacryocystorhinostomy. *Arch. Ophthalmol.* 84:765, 1970.

Verhoeff, F. H. Treatments of acute dacryocystitis. *J.A.M.A.* 60:727, 1913.

Wheeler, J. M. Removal of the lachrymal sac and accessory lachrymal gland. *Int. J. Surg.* 18:106–109, 1915.

Trauma

INJURY OF THE NASOCANTHAL ANGLE

Of the two canthi, the medial is by far the more vulnerable. It houses the puncta and delicate canaliculi which are the primary components of the tear-conducting mechanism. The vestigial plica and caruncle may be no great shakes cosmetically, but we are accustomed to them and their absence would leave the globe looking abnormally bare. When repairs are necessary the lateral canthus offers the wide-open spaces of the temporal region from which reparative tissue may be garnered. The nasocanthal angle offers only the obstructive nasal barrier that forces the surgeon to undertake much more complicated procedures.

Canalicular Tears

Probably the most common and unfortunate of nasocanthal injuries is a break in canalicular continuity. Reports of such repairs continue to baffle ophthalmologists and roil the literature. I wish I could report that recent contributions afforded improved treatment for this enigmatic and frustrating entity. But the current literature contains nothing to gladden the heart. Repair of the canalicular tear still remains an unrewarding experience for both doctor and patient. Neither the indwelling plastic tube, the metal rod, the emplaced heavy suture, nor the pigtail probe has prevented a stubborn fibrosis of the canaliculus and an almost certain obstruction of the lumen. No subject has had so many promising reports of cures exploded by the inability of others to repeat and obtain comparably brilliant results.

The one possibly hopeful fact which has emerged from this mass of discouraging literature is that the best—perhaps the only—chance for restoration of canalicular integrity lies in *early* repair. The technic of repair is not important. Technics vary with the difficulty, frequently substantial, of the repair. But unless the patient is operated on within 24 or 48 hours after injury, the repair is often doomed to failure despite assertions to the contrary in the literature. Repair is always important and should be undertaken, for a canalicular tear, no matter how severe the laceration, can often

154

be restored so that cosmetic appearance is quite acceptable. It is the functional repair which constantly eludes the ophthalmologist.

Occasionally, somewhat inexplicably, tearing ceases after repair despite a closed canaliculus. I have no explanation for this "miracle" except that drainage may continue through the upper canaliculus. In my experience upper canalicular drainage has not proved very dependable and is a weak reed to lean upon. I have seen too many eyes with patent upper and obstructed lower canaliculi which wept with undeviating persistence to the acute discomfort and embarrassment of their miserable owners. However, I have also seen more than one eye whose lower canaliculus was occluded after repair but whose owner remained uncomplaining. I can only postulate that Nature in her infinite wisdom causes a diminution in the tear secretion or that the upper canaliculus in some cases does drain off tears in sufficient quantity to keep the patient comfortable. Then why did it not work before surgery? This is not a result on which one can rely.

In the repair of torn canaliculi my success with Worst's pigtail probe has been something less than spectacular. In my hands it works sometimes; often it doesn't. It is not hard to make a false channel with the probe and never even reach the common punctum or to go around the punctum and not through it. Others have had the same experience. The difficulty, of course, is that in an old injury the medial end of the broken canaliculus remains invisible with malignant stubbornness.

It has been suggested that the upper canaliculus not be intubated in lower canalicular repair for fear that the indwelling tubing will cause injury to the upper canaliculus. It is hard to understand such reasoning. If the lower injured canaliculus can withstand intubation why cannot the intact upper? In most cases in which both canaliculi have been intubated the lower usually becomes obstructed ultimately but the upper always remains intact and patent. I do not advocate unnecessary canalicular intubation. But it frequently happens that the only way to find the medial end of the torn lower canaliculus is by way of the upper. If so, there should be no hesitancy about using the upper canaliculus.

When all other stratagems to find the medial broken end have failed, including the pigtail probe and the injection of air or milk through the upper canaliculus, only one method is reliable—retrograde passage of a probe, or better, a stiff plastic tube, from the lacrimal sac laterally to the medial opening in the broken canaliculus.

RETROGRADE CANALICULAR INTUBATION

Surgical Technic (Fig. 76): The lacrimal sac is exposed in the usual way and a 4-mm vertical incision is made in it just below the medial canthal ligament. A thin polyethylene tube* is passed through the common punctum and continued laterally and gently until it emerges through the torn medial end of the canaliculus. Since it is easy to identify the lateral end of

---

* PE 90 or PE 50.

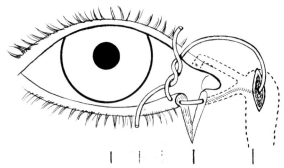

Fig. 76. Retrograde Repair of Canaliculus. Entrance to the medial end of the canalicular break is made through the opened lacrimal sac. The tubing is then pushed into the lateral end of the break, tied, and plastered to the cheek or brow.

the canalicular break, the tube is continued through to emerge from the punctum. The ends of the tubing are tied loosely and taped to the brow or cheek. The tissues of the lid around the break are carefully sutured on the conjunctival, marginal, and skin surfaces. The polyethylene tube should be left in place from 4 to 6 weeks. It is usually well tolerated.

On removal of the tube the canaliculus will remain patent for a while. But in many cases it will gradually narrow and finally close. Then recourse is to a CDCR or a combined resection of the palpebral lacrimal gland plus section of the lacrimal ductules (Chapter 9, Fig. 74).

Downward Displacement of the Medial Canthus

A rarer but more disfiguring result of nasocanthal trauma is downward displacement of the medial canthus (Fig. 77A). This may be, though not necessarily, a complication of fracture of the orbital floor, medial wall, or both. Trauma severe enough to produce this injury may also result in loss of the eye and destruction of lacrimal drainage. Depression of the medial canthus has not been reported frequently, probably not only because it is relatively uncommon but because its repair is difficult and not frequently attempted. Nevertheless, downward displacement of the medial canthus is a blemish unacceptable especially to the young. With care, it can be repaired.

REPAIR WITH TEAR DRAINAGE INTACT—AUTHOR'S METHOD

The first step is to investigate the integrity of the nasolacrimal duct by the usual means—either irrigation or a dye test. If lacrimal drainage is intact, repair proceeds as follows.

Surgical Technic (Fig. 77): After suitable anesthesia, either local or general, an incision is made as for lacrimal sac surgery. The skin and orbicularis are reflected back to disclose the anterior arm of the displaced medial

canthal ligament. This is cut close to its attachment to the maxilla and carefully freed from surrounding fibrous adhesions; a stout double-armed 3-0
or 4-0 chromic suture is passed through the cut end. The number of adhesions will depend on the severity of the causative trauma and the amount
of destruction it produced. The posterior arm of the canthal ligament is
much weaker than the anterior one and is rarely difficult to free, although
adhesions may have to be dissected away. The orbital fascia may have to
be cut above and below close to the medial orbital wall in order to mobilize
the canthus sufficiently to permit its upward rotation to a position of overcorrection, where it is sutured to the periosteum (Fig. 77B). Sometimes the
injury is so severe that the ligament itself is destroyed. In that case the
ligament must be replaced by equivalent fibrous tissue of the area which is
readily available.

When the ligament is being manipulated it is well to remember that
the canaliculi run with the anterior arm of the ligament until they enter the
lacrimal sac as the ligament crosses it. Hence care should be taken not to
injure the subjacent sac or kink the delicate canaliculi during the dissection.
If the fascial attachment to the orbital rim has been cut, it is now sutured,
and all openings into the orbit are closed. A double-armed 4-0 silk suture is
passed through the cut end of the ligament and then upward behind the
brow to emerge above the brow, where it is tied over a peg (Fig. 77C).
This position of overcorrection and the extra suture above the brow are
used to counteract the tendency for fibrous tissue healing and contraction to
pull the canthus downward again. The skin is sutured (Fig. 77D) and a
patch applied. The eye is dressed daily, the skin sutures are removed on
the fifth day and the brow sutures on the tenth day (Fig. 77E).

REPAIR WITH TEAR DRAINAGE DESTROYED—AUTHOR'S METHOD

If on investigation preoperatively the lacrimal passages are found not
to be open, there is a possibility—a slim one perhaps—that only the canaliculi are kinked. One then proceeds with the same care as described above.

When there is no functioning lacrimal drainage mechanism to preserve, the surgery is purely cosmetic and is, unfortunately, a good deal
simpler.

Surgical Technic (Fig. 78): A Z incision is made with each arm of
the incision measuring about 15 mm. The lower angle *b* of the Z encloses
the displaced canthus. The relative sizes of the upper and lower angles
depend on the amount of displacement—the greater the displacement the
larger the upper angle *a* is compared with the lower. However, one must
always keep in mind that the angles should not differ more than about 20°
or transposition will be difficult.

The two triangular skin-muscle flaps are undermined and freely
mobilized so that they may be easily transposed (Fig. 78A). This is accomplished by free incision of the orbital fascia and excision of all fibrous tissue.
If the medial canthal ligament or its surrounding tissue can be identified, it

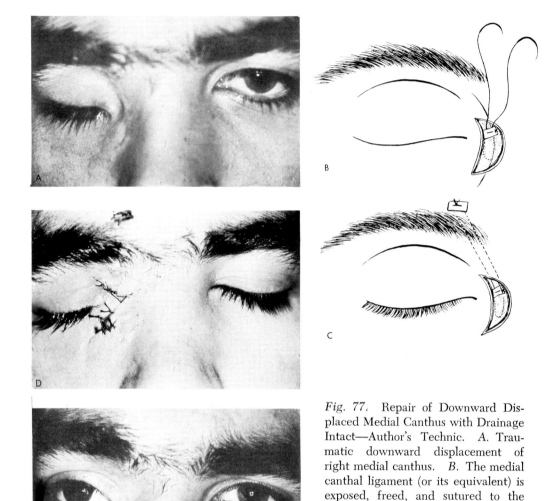

Fig. 77. Repair of Downward Displaced Medial Canthus with Drainage Intact—Author's Technic. *A.* Traumatic downward displacement of right medial canthus. *B.* The medial canthal ligament (or its equivalent) is exposed, freed, and sutured to the periosteum in a somewhat overcorrected position. *C.* The ligament is anchored by a subcutaneous suture above the brow to counteract possible downward displacement. *D.* The skin is sutured. *E.* Final result.

is freed and resutured to the medial orbital rim in a higher position. Frequently owing to the severity of the destruction it is not possible to identify the ligament, and fibrous tissue in the area may be substituted. However, this is not as important here as when lacrimal drainage has been spared. Chromic subcuticular sutures may be used to sew the flaps to the periosteum to prevent downward displacement.

The flaps *a* and *b* are transposed and the skin incisions closed with interrupted sutures of 5-0 silk (Fig. 78B). A firm supportive dressing is

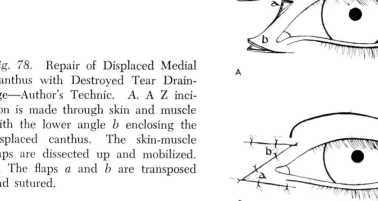

Fig. 78. Repair of Displaced Medial Canthus with Destroyed Tear Drainage—Author's Technic. A. A Z incision is made through skin and muscle with the lower angle *b* enclosing the displaced canthus. The skin-muscle flaps are dissected up and mobilized. B. The flaps *a* and *b* are transposed and sutured.

applied and postoperative care is as usual. Skin sutures are removed on the fifth or sixth postoperative day.

ORBITAL FRACTURES

The story of trauma in recent ophthalmic literature seems to be mainly the story of orbital fractures. Fractures of the orbit—especially of the orbital floor—and their complications apparently have an irresistible attraction for ophthalmologists; such reports continue to pervade the literature perhaps more than their incidence justifies. One would have thought that all that is important or germane to the subject had already been said—it probably has—but reports continue to appear.

The syndrome of serious orbital floor fracture is well known: Ptosis of the globe, enophthalmos, and supratarsal depression. There may also be diplopia, though not always. Goldstein and Greenstein have shown that there is no diplopia as long as the visual axes remain parallel.

The surgical approach to blowout fractures is standardized and is well covered in the literature of the past few years. The injured orbit is best entered at the lower orbital rim where it is most accessible and least vulnerable to surgical insult. Butler *et al.* suggest combining the usual transcutaneous infraorbital approach with antrotomy in cases where the orbital rim has also been fractured.

When or whether to operate is not as well established. However, it seems fairly evident that the tendency to operate as soon as the diagnosis of blowout fracture is established is not as attractive as it was several years ago. More and more, ophthalmic surgeons feel that a small orbital floor fracture with no obvious symptoms and normal ocular motility does not constitute an urgent indication for surgery. Edema and hemorrhage may render duction tests misleading for the first few days after blowout fracture. Hence these should be postponed until several days after injury.

Emery and his coworkers report that diplopia associated with orbital fracture often disappears in 2 weeks. For this reason they make no move to correct a blowout fracture unless there is an extensive orbital floor defect or diplopia has not disappeared in 2 weeks. In their series patients have done at least as well without surgical interference as with it. They conclude that hypocycloidal polytomography is the most accurate x-ray technic currently available for diagnosing orbital floor fractures.

After the effects of trauma such as edema and hemorrhage subside and enophthalmos with ptosis of the globe develops, surgical exploration is indicated. Of course, in a large fracture of the orbital floor associated with obvious ptosis of the globe which cannot be raised by forced duction, entrance into the orbit is necessary to free incarcerated muscle and other orbital tissues. In such a case long postponement of correction jeopardizes the chances for restoration of function or even for a decent cosmetic result.

Repair of the orbital floor is usually not difficult unless destruction is so vast that not enough floor remains to support the reparative material. Here a suggestion by Wilkins and Callahan is ingenious. They wedge a silicone block into the maxillary sinus to act as a support for the orbital contents. Various types of inert alloplastic materials are being used now. One of the most recent is the Dacron-mesh-based implant suggested by Browning. All these materials work well as long as repair is not too long postponed—i.e., after original hemorrhage and edema have subsided. These technics are well reported in the ophthalmic literature.

Enophthalmos and Supratarsal Depression

These unholy twins are common complications of blowout fractures and usually go hand in hand in severe injury. Unless the orbital floor fracture is repaired before orbital contents atrophy and shrink, the globe will become displaced not only downward but backward, producing not only ptosis of the globe but also enophthalmos and a deep depression above the tarsus of the uper lid (Fig. 79A). The depression can usually be corrected by early repair of the orbital floor and restoration of contents which have dropped into the sinus (Fig. 79B).

A supratarsal sulcus may result not only from the ptosis of the globe and hence loss of its support to the lid, but also from a drooping of the superior rectus muscle with a consequent pulling down of the levator (since both have a common anlage). Soll has suggested placement of a silicone balloon prosthesis under the periosteum of the orbital floor to lift the artificial eye and thus correct the supratarsal sulcus. This does not suffice in old injuries; these require implantation of various materials to fill the depression.

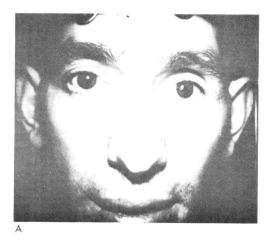

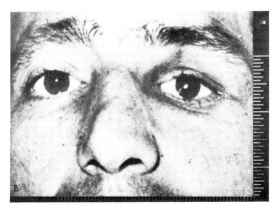

Fig. 79. Repair of Supratarsal Depression. *A.* Appearance of the left eye before repair. *B.* Appearance after repair of orbital floor fracture.

Enophthalmos may be due to incarceration of the inferior rectus in the floor fracture. Hence the orbital floor should always be inspected and the muscle released at the time of the initial repair of the fracture.

"Blowout" fracture as originally defined referred to fracture of the orbital floor only. In the literature it has been used—probably misused—to refer to all types of orbital fractures. Such reports should be scanned carefully for description of the symptoms and their sources. For example, when symptoms include subcutaneous emphysema, epistaxis, and downward displacement of the medial canthus (Fig. 77A), fracture of the medial orbital wall should be suspected rather than a true blowout. In this case retraction of the globe may be due to incarceration of the medial rectus muscle.

All orbital fractures, including the blowout fracture, range from mild to extremely severe; many can be serious indeed. Fradkin, who reported 61 orbital fractures, found that almost all were associated with lid, conjunctival, and muscle damage. But, more serious, 40 per cent were associated with ocular injuries of major severity, including rupture of the globe, intraocular hemorrhage, cataract, choroidal rupture, and optic nerve damage. Only 12 of his 61 patients did not require surgery.

Not much has been said about the affect of orbital fracture repair on visual acuity. But recent reports have shown that vision can be severely compromised as the result of orbital floor surgery. In a review of 72 patients whose orbital floor fractures were repaired with silicone subperiosteal implants, Nicholson and Guzak reported that 6 suffered subsequent visual loss. In 2 cases vision was restored by removal of the implant. In the other 4 the loss, either partial or complete, was permanent.

COMPLICATIONS OF THE ANOPHTHALMIC SOCKET

Enophthalmos and supratarsal depression in an anophthalmic socket produce disfigurement that requires correction. Sometimes these conditions are present almost immediately; occasionally they appear years after enucleation. Late-appearing disfigurement may result from the use of a too small ball implant originally, from migration of an implant, or from absorption of the implant if organic material was used. Even years later, these untoward developments can be alleviated by increasing orbital contents. Since the orbit is a cone-shaped area with the only opening in front, anything that fills the orbit will tend to push a prosthesis forward and hence decrease enophthalmos.

DELAYED IMPLANT—AUTHOR'S METHOD

In the past almost every conceivable organic material has been tried. Today's surgeon uses the new inert plastic substances which are easily manageable and do well. No matter what the material or shape of the implant, it must be well covered and must not overfill the orbit.

Surgical Technic (Fig. 80): A horizontal incision is made in the fundus of the socket and the conjunctiva undermined upward and downward to expose Tenon's capsule. The capsule is entered through a small horizontal incision and the opening enlarged with a large Kelly clamp to make ample room for the implant (Fig. 80A). The implant is inserted. Whatever the shape or material of the implant, ample room must be created for it so that it can be inserted easily without the slightest forcing. A solid methyl methacrylate ball or the smaller Pyrex beads (Fig. 80B) may be preferred; all work well.

A pursestring or crossed-sutures closure with 4-0 chromic catgut is made in Tenon's capsule (Fig. 80C). After closure, search is made for any lesser openings and additional single-armed sutures are used to seal the wound completely. The conjunctiva is drawn over and closed horizontally

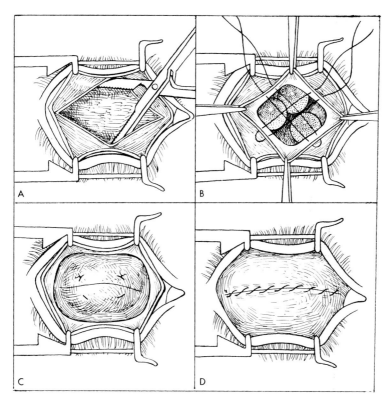

Fig. 80. Insertion of Delayed Implant into Tenon's Capsule. *A.* The conjunctival sac is opened widely; Tenon's capsule is incised horizontally and entered with forceps, and the opening enlarged. *B.* The desired implant is inserted (glass beads in this case). *C.* Tenon's capsule is tightly closed by crossed sutures. *D.* The conjunctiva is closed with a running suture.

with a running suture of 6-0 silk (Fig. 80*D*). A conformer is inserted and a pressure dressing applied and kept on for 5 days to assure healing with the implant in proper position.

Comment: For some time I have preferred the Berens implant, shaped like a truncated cone. This comes in several sizes and conforms to the cone shape of the orbit. I feel that it retains its position better than a glass ball. Occasionally when correcting enophthalmos caused by too small an implant, I have not bothered to remove the original well-embedded material, but have simply inserted another implant of the same size or somewhat larger over it. This works out quite well provided, again, that the implant fits in easily and without pressure.

A word of caution. The socket should not be made so shallow as to prevent the insertion of a decent-sized prosthesis. I have seen this happen in secondary socket reconstructions with a cosmetic result almost as bad as the condition which required repair originally. Sufficient depth should be left for insertion of a reform prosthesis rather than a shell, which is less acceptable cosmetically.

Results of such operations are not always perfect but they do a great deal—sometimes enough—to alleviate the disfigurement.

REPLACEMENT OF AN EXTRUDED IMPLANT

Enucleations are done less frequently as our ability to save eyes improves. But if recent literature is any criterion, the extruded implant is still a complication to be reckoned with.

The implant has gone through a long series of evolutions since the Second World War—from the buried sphere to the integrated sphere to the semiintegrated sphere and back to the buried sphere. (Some of these "spheres" have had curious aspherical shapes.)

No matter how careful the surgery, a certain percentage of the implants—glass, gold, plastic—will extrude. Replacement always involves loss of conjunctival tissue, a smaller implant, a supratarsal depression, and sometimes enophthalmos. In 1967 Iliff made an ingenious suggestion. He replaced an extruded implant with a hollow silicone air-filled sphere introduced through a lateral brow incision. He thus avoided not only passing the implant through possibly infected areas but also the inevitable shortening of conjunctiva following incision. Beyer and Smith use small 5-mm Pyrex beads to replace an extruded implant (Fig. 80B). Helveston prefers scleral patching to repair the opening in Tenon's capsule rather than replacing the implant. He uses fresh or preserved sclera and reports excellent results.

OCCULT EYE PERFORATIONS

A recent report by Goldberg and Tessler has little to do with lid surgery but does deal with lid trauma. It is of importance for the ophthalmic surgeon. The authors point out that minor brow and lid lacerations caused by narrow, sharp objects such as darts, scissors, and fine knives may mask unsuspected associated scleral and retinal perforations even though these structures are apparently remote from the site of primary injury. Furthermore, the classic signs of scleral perforation—lid edema, chemosis, perilimbal hyperemia, lacrimation, hypotony, and vitreous hemorrhage—may not always be present. Hence they recommend the following regimen whenever a scleral perforation is considered possible: (1) immediate pupillary dilation and complete ocular examination including fundus, under general anesthesia if necessary; (2) sedation and bed rest if a scleral perforation is found; (3) surgical exploration, even in doubtful cases, and repair of scleral and retinal tears if found.

REFERENCES

Beyer, C. K. and Smith, B. Glass bead implants. *Arch. Ophthalmol.* 82:214, 1969.

Browning, C. W. Dacron mesh-based implants for orbital floor reconstructions. *Am. J. Ophthalmol.* 68:914, 1969.

Butler, R. M., Morledge, D., Holt, J. P., Kreiger, A. E. A system of surgical approaches to orbital floor fractures. *Trans. Am. Acad. Ophthalmol. Otolaryngol.* 75:519, 1971.

Emery, J. M., von Noorden, G. K., and Schlernitzauer, D. A. Orbital floor fractures: Long-term follow-up of cases with and without surgical repair. *Trans. Am. Acad. Ophthalmol. Otolaryngol.* 75:802, 1971.

Fox, S. A. Downward displacement of the medial canthus. *Ann. Ophthalmol.* 3:1082, 1971.

Fradkin, A. H. Orbital floor fractures and ocular complications. *Am. J. Ophthalmol.* 72:699, 1971.

Goldberg, M. F., and Tessler, H. H. Occult intraocular perforations from brow and lid lacerations. *Arch. Ophthalmol.* 86:145, 1971.

Goldstein, J. H., and Greenstein, V. Absence of diplopia in ptosis of the globe. *Ann. Ophthalmol.* 2:373, 1970.

Helveston, E. M. A scleral patch for exposed implants. *Trans. Am. Acad. Ophthalmol. Otolaryngol.* 74:1307, 1970.

Iliff, C. E. The extruded implant. *Arch. Ophthalmol.* 78:742, 1967.

Nicholson, D. H., and Guzak, S. V. Visual loss complicating repair of orbital floor fractures. *Arch. Ophthalmol.* 86:369, 1971.

Robinson, T. J., and Strang, M. F. The anatomy of the medial canthal ligament. *Br. J. Plast. Surg.* 23:1, 1970.

Smith, B. C., Barr, D. R., and Langham, E. J. Complication of orbital fracture. *N.Y. State J. Med.* 71:2407, 1971.

Soll, D. B. Correction of superior lid sulcus with periosteal implants. *Arch. Ophthalmol.* 85:188, 1971.

Wilkins, R. B., and Callahan, A. Repair of enophthalmic anophthalmos. *Am. J. Ophthalmol.* 68:936, 1969.

Worst, J. G. F. Method of reconstructing torn lacrimal canaliculus. *Am. J. Ophthalmol.* 53:520, 1962.

Index